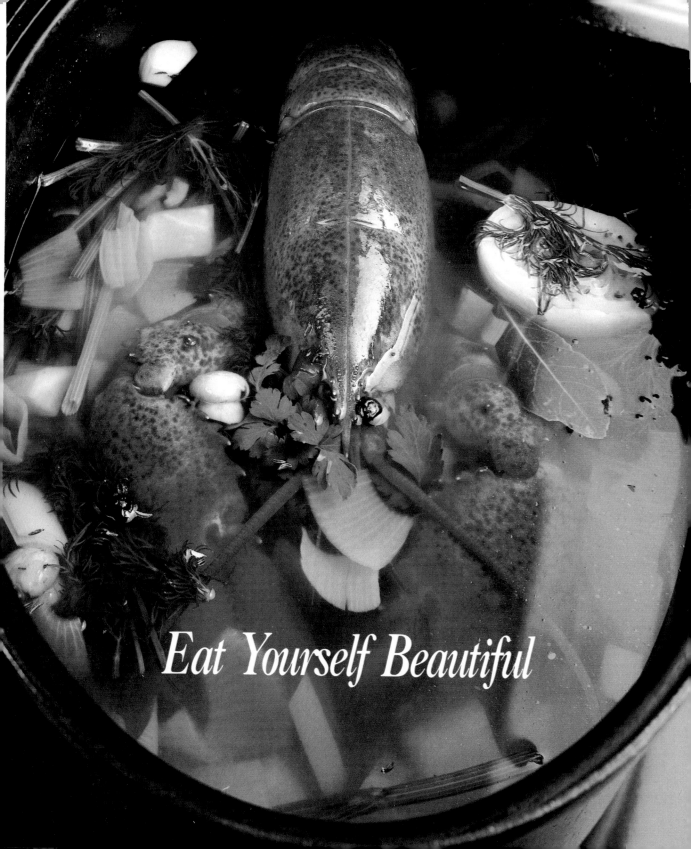

Eat Yourself Beautiful

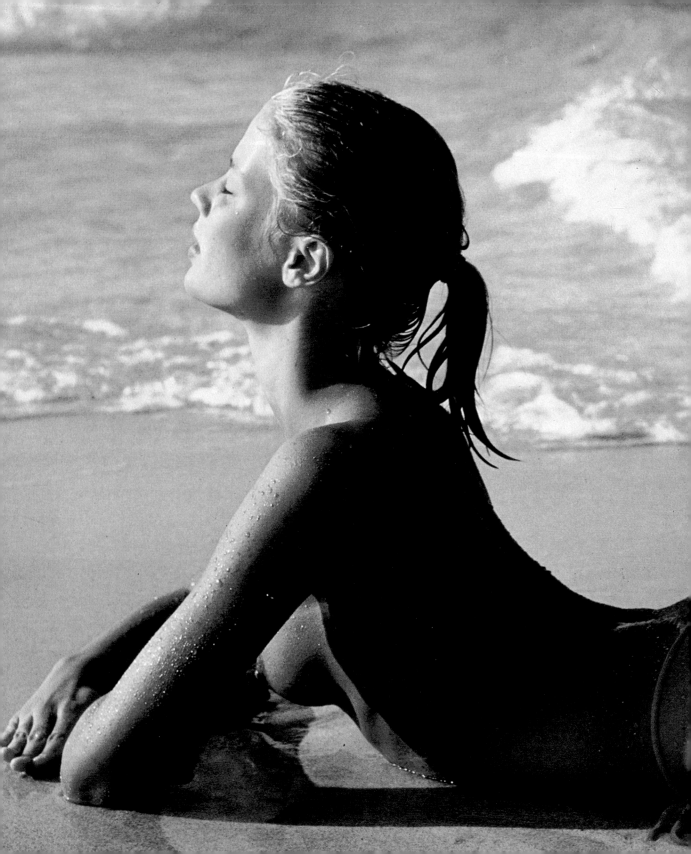

Eat Yourself Beautiful

Your Strategy for Lifelong Beauty

Daniele de Winter

Foreword by Jan de Winter, M.D.

Translated from German by Else Daniels

ACROPOLIS BOOKS LTD.

WASHINGTON, D.C.

Translated from German by Else Daniel

Eat Yourself Beautiful published and copyright 1986 by Verlag Michael Lechner, Vienna, Austria.

Cover photo: Carolyn Stuckey;
Other photos: ZEFA, Vienna, Austria

ACROPOLIS BOOKS, LTD.
Colortone Building, 2400 17th St., N.W., Washington, D.C. 20009

Printed in the United States of America by
COLORTONE PRESS
Creative Graphics, Inc.
Washington, D.C. 20009

Attention: Schools and Corporations
ACROPOLIS books are available at quantity discounts with bulk purchase for educational, business, or sales promotional use. For information, please write to: SPECIAL SALES DEPARTMENT, ACROPOLIS BOOKS LTD., 2400 17th ST., N.W., WASHINGTON, D.C. 20009

Are there Acropolis Books you want but cannot find in your local stores?
You can get any Acropolis book title in print. Simply send title and retail price, plus $1.50 per copy to cover mailing and handling costs for each book desired. District of Columbia residents add applicable sales tax. Enclose check or money order only, no cash please, to: ACROPOLIS BOOKS LTD., 2400 17th St., N.W., WASHINGTON, D.C. 20009

Library of Congress Cataloging-in-Publication Data
De Winter, Daniele, 1963–
    Eat yourself beautiful.

    Includes index.
    1. Nutrition. 2. Beauty, Personal. I. Title.
RA784.D43 1987 613.2 87-1431
ISBN 0-87491-860-X (pbk.)

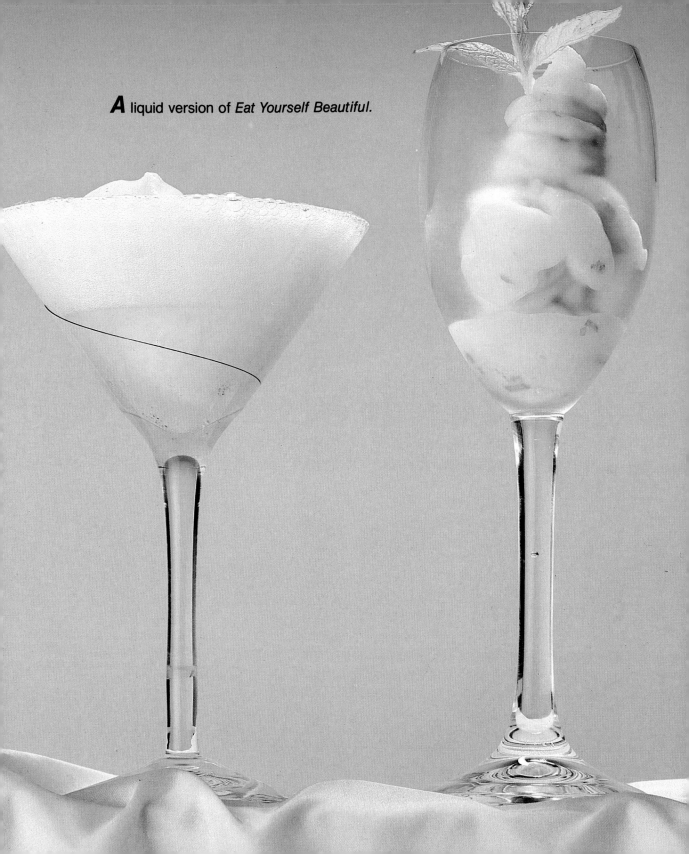

A liquid version of *Eat Yourself Beautiful.*

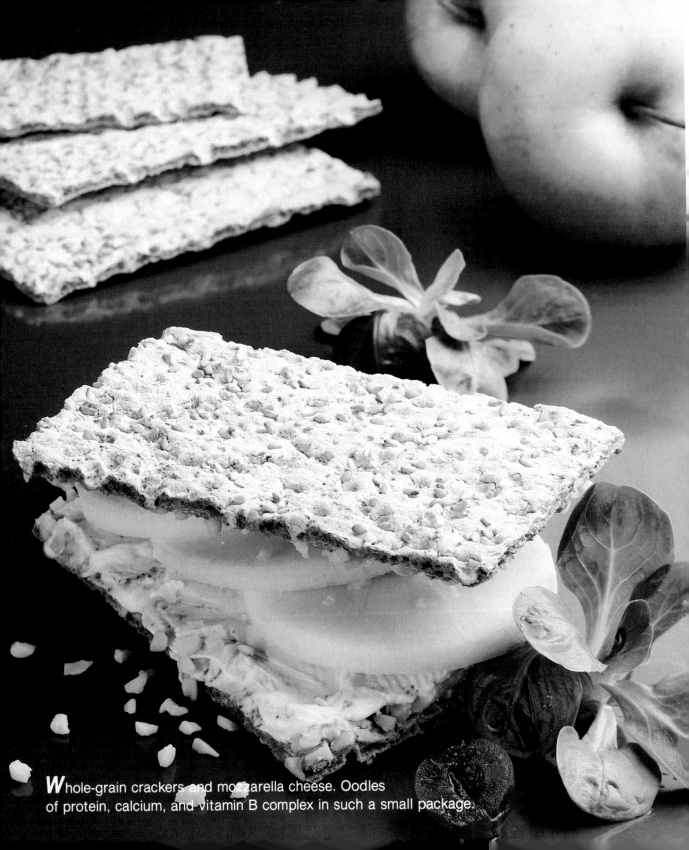

Whole-grain crackers and mozzarella cheese. Oodles of protein, calcium, and vitamin B complex in such a small package.

C O N T E N T S

EAT YOURSELF BEAUTIFUL

Feeling glamorous has a galvanizing effect on the immune system, which protects the body against disease. Therefore, women should always strive to look their best, not only for reasons of vanity but also to maintain good health. Daniele de Winter's book *EAT YOURSELF BEAUTIFUL* makes a valuable contribution to the advancement of public education in health and should be read by all women.

My daughter Daniele is qualified to write on the significant influence that sensible eating can exert on a woman's appearance because of her nutritional expertise, which she acquired during her prolonged apprenticeship as my assistant. She also has a second great asset: she is a very experienced, competent, and innovative cook.

Furthermore, because Daniele is a woman, she knows what goes on in a woman's mind, particularly with regard to stress, aging, and the transient nature of beauty.

This book is very reassuring to those who suffer from constant self-doubt. It is full of common sense and practical advice on all facets of living, including such vital aspects as regular exercise and control of stress.

A large selection of mouth-watering food tips have been included for all times of the day, and countless culinary delights are suggested for special occasions. All the dishes are inexpensive as well as easy to prepare; they are invariably nutritious, rich in fiber, and nonfattening.

For the woman who wants to continue looking youthful and feeling her best, this scientifically sound and extremely readable book is an absolute must.

Jan de Winter, MD, FRCR, FFR, RCSI, ADMR

What Does EAT YOURSELF BEAUTIFUL Mean?

Suppose there were a way to live up to your full beauty potential, to make the very most of what nature has given you. Suppose you could make your hair its most lustrous, your skin its most radiant, your eyes their sparkliest, and that all of these beautiful traits reflected your body at its very best. Imagine how happy you would be to look so good and feel so well because you're so happy. Then smile and pat yourself on the back, because by thinking this way you've just created a "beauty circle." That's what this book is all about.

A beauty circle is the exact opposite of a vicious circle. In the vicious circle you go round and round pushed by negative feelings, which are hard to interrupt. In the beauty circle you do good things for yourself that make you beautiful. The pleasure, the happy feeling, you get from being beautiful makes you feel good and that good feeling keeps the circle going to again make you beautiful and glamorous. Seems like magic and in a way it is—think about the original meaning of the word glamor, it comes from the old English word *gramarye,* which means magic, to cast a spell. While there's a logical explanation for this particular magic, the results are so marvelous that it might seem a little unreal at first.

Beauty circle magic is connected very closely with your health. Recent research shows that happiness actually has a beneficial effect on your immune system, which fights off diseases and keeps you healthy. Your beauty circle is not a frivolous idea that will have people shaking their heads and muttering about vanity. Your beauty circle has everything to do with keeping you well physically and emotionally, enabling you to function effectively, accomplish what you set for yourself, and enjoy it all.

Here's where *Eat Yourself Beautiful* comes in. It actually starts your beauty circle and keeps it going. *Eat Yourself Beautiful* is an approach to eating based on the idea that there is a direct and absolute relationship between the foods we eat and how we look and feel. That in turn is based on nutritional research that has been conducted for years at the de Winter Clinic for Cancer Prevention Advice in England where I worked with my father, Dr. Jan de Winter, developing the *Eat Yourself Beautiful* approach.

This is a simple, no-nonsense approach based on a great variety of foods and promoting well-balanced, delicious eating. It's an attitude toward eating where you consistently choose what's best for you and leave out what's harmful. What's best for you and why is something you're going to find out in the first chapter of this book. You might think of this as effective eating, because everything you eat works to make you beautiful and healthy.

Moreover, because the "beauty foods" are so appealing, it's easy to make this food approach into a lifelong beauty and health strategy. There are no hard and fast rules; no one thinks that you can or should live on a diet of boiled lentil skins mixed with desiccated liver. It wouldn't even be good for you! This is a relaxed approach that recognizes the pleasure and aesthetics of eating (check out the tempting pictures), and that recognition is exactly what makes it easy to follow. That—and the results, being as beautiful as you can be—is pretty irresistible. In addition, knowing that you're doing yourself so much good makes beginning your beauty circle with *Eat Yourself Beautiful* a top priority.

Daniele de Winter

BEAUTY FOODS: What Are They?

Beauty Foods can work the magic! They are the ones with the nutrients, vitamins, and minerals that have a direct effect on your entire system. Vitamins and minerals are organic substances that our bodies cannot make for the most part, and that we have to acquire from what we eat. The trick is to select the foods that contain the right balance of these nutrients, because if you skimp on any, your body will let you know.

The foods that provide the highest concentration are those we think of as "beauty foods." They are the natural, fresh, and unrefined products we talk about in this book, and they are the foods we'd like to encourage you to eat more of. We've provided recipes in Chapter Two that use lots of beauty foods in appealing dishes. But before you turn to these, you'll want some information about the vitamins and minerals themselves. To make it easier and to show you at a glance where you can find the beauty components, we've included a chart at the end of the chapter that lists many of the foods that contain these components. You'll learn how they affect your body.

Once you realize that increasing your beauty vitamin intake can give your dry, greasy, or muddy-looking skin a dewy radiance and that increasing the amount of whole grains you eat can make your dull hair gleam, then you can take charge. You have the means to live up to your beauty potential right on your own grocery list. And not just your external beauty potential. Providing your body with the beauty food components keeps your entire system in balance. At the most regular level, your mental and emotional well-being are directly affected by the regular intake of certain vitamins.

Vitamins and minerals are the building blocks of all the complex mechanisms that insure the body's metabolic function. Vitamins, after all, were so named because "vita" means life. Each makes its contribution to our well-being, but the key is that they work together.

Beauty Vitamins

VITAMIN A: Vitamin A is involved in the body's growth and healing processes and is also needed for good vision, especially at night. It is one of the major skin vitamins because it plays an active role in the metabolism of the skin cells. It helps to slough off dry cells and therefore keeps skin soft and smooth. Vitamin A protects the skin against dryness and premature aging (i.e., the formation of wrinkles and the development of irregular pigmentation). A proper supply of vitamin A also guards the skin against infection.

According to Dr. George Wolf, a nutritionist at the Massachusetts Institute of Technology, vitamin A is an anti-infection vitamin because it strengthens walls of skin cells, making them less susceptible to penetration by microorganisms.

Vitamin A is found chiefly in green and yellow vegetables, and in milk, eggs, liver, fish-liver oils, and many fruits.

B-COMPLEX VITAMINS:
The B-complex vitamins are essential for a properly functioning nervous system and for maintaining healthy skin and hair. Vitamin B is the "Big-Beauty B." It simply helps everything. It nourishes your skin, and soothes away tension lines. Too little vitamin B results in skin problems, lip hair, fatigue, nervousness, and even depression.

There are more than ten B vitamins. While they have specific individual functions, they occur together in many of the same foods and work together as an efficient team.

For example, Vitamin B_2 (riboflavin) is essential for strong, lustrous hair and healthy skin. It helps your body to convert carbohydrates, proteins, and fats into energy. A B_2 deficiency shows up in the form of dull, oily skin, hair loss, hypersensitive areas around the nose and mouth, a tendency to pimples, and hypersensitivity of the eyes.

Vitamin B_6 (pyridoine) is necessary for the production of collagen and elastin, which keep your skin smooth and maintain its elasticity.

You might think of B_6 as the anti-aging vitamin. An adequate supply of B_6 protects you against eczema, dandruff, and other skin problems that interfere with looking your best.

Another B vitamin that is important to good looks is vitamin B_{12} (cobalamin), which protects against anemia, helping you to look healthy and have good color.

In order to get enough of the B vitamins, make sure you eat whole-grain products, yeast-rich foods, wheat germ, fresh fruits and vegetables, liver, nuts, and dairy products.

VITAMIN C:

Vitamin C is probably the most important vitamin for maintaining health and beauty. Vitamin C is essential to the production of collagen, the connective tissue that holds cells together. Because of its role in producing collagen, this vitamin promotes smooth and elastic skin. Vitamin C helps to prevent wrinkles and is also used very successfully for the treatment of acne, eczema, and other skin problems.

In addition to maintaining the skin, vitamin C helps to develop healthy blood vessels, to form the dentine layer of your teeth, to harden bones, and to heal burns and wounds. It strengthens the immune system and protects against colds, infections, and painful swollen joints.

The best sources of vitamin C are citrus fruits of all kinds, leafy green vegetables, peppers, tomatoes, and blueberries. It is present in all fresh fruits and vegetables to some degree.

VITAMIN D:

We need vitamin D for strong bones and teeth and for good vision. It is also necessary for proper processing of calcium and phosphorus.

The body actually makes its own vitamin D when exposed to the sun. But, since beautiful skin demands that your exposure to the sun should be limited, you can get vitamin D from fortified milk; certain fatty fish (like tuna and salmon); and fish-liver oils, egg yolks, and liver.

VITAMIN E:

Like vitamins A, B, and C, vitamin E is also essential for lasting beauty. This vitamin increases the oxygen intake of cells, which allows faster healing and regeneration. In connection with exercise, vitamin E aids muscle development. It also helps to prevent varicose veins; large quantities of vitamin E are used to treat varicose veins.

Vitamin E is present in wheat germ, seeds and whole-grain products, cold-pressed vegetable oils (olive and sunflower), green leafy vegetables, as well as eggs.

VITAMIN K:

While vitamin K does not appear to have a direct effect on appearance, it is absolutely essential for proper blood clotting and helps to maintain normal bone metabolism. Doctors increasingly believe that vitamin K keeps you younger longer because it provides energy for your cells.

Eat yoghurt, milk, and eggs to maintain your vitamin K supply, as well as leafy green vegetables, liver, and cereals. Vitamin K is also found in fish-liver oil.

FATTY ACIDS:

Fatty acids are not official vitamins, but since they help to promote proper skin metabolism, the process of forming and sloughing cells at the right speed and in the right amounts, they are included here. Fatty acids are necessary for beautiful skin and properly functioning glands and mucous membranes. You shouldn't ever eliminate unsaturated fatty acids from your diet, even when you're trying to reduce your fat intake. A lack of these substances will become apparent very quickly, because your hair will be dry and you may develop dandruff, your nails will be brittle, and your skin will lose its radiance.

The body cannot form these fatty acids, so you'll have to get them from your food. Nibble nuts and seeds (like sunflower and pumpkin), sprinkle wheat germ on your cereal, use a little butter. Vitamin F also occurs in lecithin and fish-liver oil.

Beauty Minerals

Now let's consider the beauty minerals that you need to maintain good looks and good health. Certain minerals are essential for the development of healthy skin, muscles, blood, bones, and nerves. And, of course, your body's good health will be reflected in your glowing skin and gleaming hair.

As is true of the vitamins, there are certain minerals that are especially important to maintaining good looks. These beauty minerals are calcium, copper, iodine, iron, potassium, sulfur, selenium, and zinc. Other minerals, such as chromium, fluorine, magnesium, manganese, molybdenum, nickel, phosphorus, silicon, strontium, tin, and vanadium are important for a healthy body, but they do not appear to have any particular effect on our appearance (except for fluoride, which will make teeth less susceptible to cavities when used on a regular basis).

CALCIUM: Like vitamin A, calcium is a must for healthy skin. It is important for our overall well-being because we use it every day for many bodily functions. It promotes strong bones and teeth and a healthy heart. Calcium is involved in the transmission of nerve impulses and in the contraction of muscles.

Calcium is very important for everyone, but it is especially important for women after menopause. If you don't have enough calcium, your bones will become brittle and have a tendency to break at the slightest impact. This condition is known as osteoporosis and, while it can affect everyone, women are afflicted more often than men. It's a condition you should and can guard against by making sure that you get enough calcium, starting at an early age. If your food doesn't provide an adequate supply, your body will try to maintain a proper level of the mineral by taking it out of your bones. It's an insidious process and it makes your bones fragile long before anything shows up on x rays. So, to prevent your bones from softening, make sure that your calcium intake is adequate.

Calcium is found in all dairy products, in green leafy vegetables, in whole grains, and in certain fish, such as salmon and sardines. The bones of these fish are a superb source of calcium. They're so soft that you can crush them up when you're making salmon salad or a sardine hors d'oeuvre.

COPPER: Copper is important to beauty because it helps to maintain natural hair color and keeps skin elastic. It is involved in the development of red blood cells and is needed for the proper formation of respiratory enzymes.

Copper is found in whole-grain products, fish and seafood, yeast, and liver. Practically no one in the developed countries has a copper deficiency, because there are minute quantities in our tap water.

IODINE: According to Leslie Kenton, nutritional editor for *Harper & Queens* magazine, iodine is important for beautiful hair. It keeps hair strong and glossy and protects against rough and wrinkled skin. We also need iodine for our metabolism and to regulate our energy supply. We can satisfy our iodine requirement by eating fish and seafood and even, occasionally, seaweed (kelp).

IRON: Iron strengthens our hair and nails. An inadequate supply of iron makes us pale, weak, and extremely sensitive to cold. A proper iron supply promotes healthy red blood, which is reflected in proper skin color.

Iron is present in egg yolks, liver, and red meat, green leafy vegetables (remember Popeye and the instant energy he got from a can of spinach), whole-grain products, and fish. Cooking in cast-iron pots also adds iron to your diet.

POTASSIUM: Potassium protects against dry skin and blemishes. It maintains the body's acid-base equilibrium. Potassium is essential to the production of energy and it also helps in the removal of waste materials (through bowel movements) which helps to keep our skin looking clear.

Potassium is found in citrus fruits and bananas, many vegetables, fish, meat, and in all whole-grain products.

SULFUR: Sulfur is essential for lasting beauty because it keeps skin, hair, and nails healthy. Very often, a lack of sulfur in the diet is the cause of brittle nails. Sulfur is present in fish, eggs, beef, and some vegetables, especially the cabbage family and onions.

SELENIUM: Selenium helps to keep skin young-looking and elastic. It is found in eggs, brewer's yeast, onions, garlic, and tuna.

SILICON: Silicon is another skin smoother. It also makes your nails strong and your hair glossy. Eat apples, avocados, and honey to fill your silicon requirement.

ZINC: Zinc is also important for lovely skin. Like the B vitamins and sulfur, it is involved in collagen production, and collagen contributes to supple, elastic skin. Because zinc helps to maintain the elasticity of your skin, it can help prevent stretch marks on your stomach and hips. You might think of it as the anti-sag mineral.

Zinc is also necessary for good digestion and for insuring a good oxygen supply for every part of the body. Again, like the B vitamins, it is active in the growth and healing processes.

We can get zinc from whole-grain products, nuts, legumes, oysters, and meat.

Fiber—A Beauty Bonus
Known to Our Grandmothers

In addition to vitamins and minerals, which have such obvious effects on our beauty, there is another beauty substance you'll want to know about. It's a non-nutrient that our grandmothers used to call roughage, i.e., the fibrous portion of food that is not digested and that is eliminated by the organism in approximately the same form in which it's ingested.

We consider it a beauty bonus for the following reasons:

- Fiber itself contains no calories. So, when you eat food with a high-fiber content, it doesn't pad your total caloric intake—or you.

- Your stomach and small intestine work harder to separate digestible material from indigestible dietary fiber. This slow digestion insures an even flow of calories, which keeps you from feeling hungry for longer periods.

- Once the indigestible fiber has been separated out in the stomach and small intestine, it passes through the large intestine very quickly, which causes the rapid elimination of waste products. The result of this rapid elimination, or short transit time, is clear skin, sparkling eyes, and a feeling of well-being.

Rapid elimination of waste products is now also thought to provide some protection against bowel and colon cancer. The shorter the transit time of waste material through the large intestine, the less time there is for the formation of toxic substances that are thought to be carcinogenic, or cancer-producing.

Fiber is found in all raw vegetables and fruits and in natural grains. The outer layers of grains such as oats, wheat, and sesame consist primarily of fiber; they also contain more vitamins and minerals than the inner layers. Dr. Jan de Winter, director of the Cancer Prevention Foundation in England and the author's father, says: "We could live by bread alone—provided it's whole-grain. It has protein and complex carbohydrates and could form the basis of our diet. . . . It takes eight white loaves to produce the fiber content of one whole-grain loaf."

Since the beauty foods consist chiefly of raw vegetables and fruits, whole grains, nuts, and seeds, they also supply the body with the necessary fiber.

THE BEAUTY FOODS SHOPPING LIST

Fill your grocery cart with these Beauty Foods and you'll soon glow with good health.

Fruits

apples	lemons
apricots	melons
avocados	oranges
bananas	pears
blueberries	pineapple
cherries	raisins
coconut	raspberries
currants	strawberries
grapes	tangerines
kiwis	tomatoes

Vegetables

cabbage	mushrooms
carrots	olives
celery	onions
cucumbers	peppers—all colors
eggplant	potatoes
kohlrabi	radicchio
leeks	scallions
lettuce—all kinds	spinach
	watercress

Meats, Fish, Poultry, Eggs

beef, lean
chicken
eggs

fish—all kinds
shrimp
turkey

Breads

whole-grain

Dairy Products

buttermilk
low-fat milk (enriched with
  vitamin A and D)
cottage cheese (low fat)

mozzarella
Parmesan cheese
yoghurt (low fat)
frozen yoghurt (low fat)

Nuts & Seeds

almonds
walnuts
all sprouts and seeds

sesame seeds
pumpkin seeds
sunflower seeds

Pasta

all kinds—whole grain

Whole Grains

bran	rice, brown
oats	flour, unbleached

Seasonings

basil	all polyunsaturated oils
chives	mustard, Dijon
dill	olive oil
garlic	parsley
honey	sea salt
low cholesterol cooking	sunflower oil
spray	thyme
mint	vinegar

Vitamins and Minerals:
Where They're Found and What They Do

Vitamin or mineral	Some of the foods in which it's found	What it's good for
Vitamin A	cheeses, eggs, yoghurt, butter, margarine, crab, oysters, salmon, swordfish, tuna, bananas, peaches, apricots, nectarines, chicken, broccoli, cabbage, carrots, chives, asparagus, watercress, lettuces, red peppers, peas, squash, sweet potatoes, pumpkin, spinach, all forms of tomato	beautiful skin vision (especially at night) guards against infection
Vitamin B-complex	whole-wheat flour, oatmeal, wheat germ, brown rice, soybean products, dried beans and peas, brewer's yeast, almonds, pecans, walnuts, avocados, beef, mushrooms, peanuts, turkey, veal, pork, canned tuna, cheeses, skim milk, yoghurt	beautiful skin glorious hair healthy nervous system helps release energy from carbohydrates, fats, and protein
Vitamin C	oranges, lemons, limes, pineapples, strawberries, cantaloupe, tomatoes, green peppers, broccoli, blueberries, Brussels sprouts, kale, calves' liver	collagen formation elastic skin prevention of wrinkles immune system

Vitamin D	fortified milk, egg yolks, liver, tuna, salmon, cod-liver oil, sunshine	strong bones and teeth healthy eyes involved in calcium/ phosphorus metabolism
Vitamin E	vegetable oils, wheat germ, avocados, butter, roasted peanuts, broiled salmon, whole-grain cereals, cabbage, spinach	may increase healing protects vitamin A and essential fatty acids from oxidation
Unsaturated fatty acids	wheat germ, margarine, lecithin, nuts, sunflower and pumpkin seeds, avocados	skin metabolism
Vitamin K	yoghurt, milk, eggs, spinach, kale, cabbage, cauliflower, liver, potatoes, peas, whole-grain cereals	proper blood clotting normal bone metabolism
Calcium	milk, cheese, yoghurt, mussels, sardines, clams, oysters, dates, almonds, broccoli, chickpeas, rhubarb	strong bones and teeth transmission of nerve impulses prevention of osteoporosis relaxing

Copper	oysters, cherries, cocoa powder, chicken, dried beans, kidneys, nuts, liver, drinking water	maintains hair color elastic skin red blood cells respiratory enzymes
Iodine	fish, oysters, kelp, sea salt, shrimp	beautiful hair thyroid metabolism beautiful skin
Iron	egg yolks, liver, molasses, peaches, apricots, prunes, raisins, shrimp, whole-grain breads, red meats	red blood cells hair nails
Potassium	bran, rye wafers, raisins, pecans, dried peaches, orange juice, bananas, potatoes, almonds, dried apricots	acid-base balance body water balance
Sulfur	eggs, beef, wheat germ, dried beans and peas, peanuts, clams, cabbage, onions	beautiful skin, hair, and nails
Selenium	meat, egg yolks, chicken, garlic, onions, tuna, brewer's yeast	elastic skin works with vitamin E

Silicon	apples, avocados, honey, nuts	beautiful skin, hair, and nails
Zinc	wheat germ, brewer's yeast, herring, seafood, liver, milk, eggs	good digestion good oxygen supply to all parts of body growth and healing

Beauty Food Recipes

The previous chapter discussed the beauty benefits of individual vitamins and minerals and where they're found. Now, we're going to be more specific and show you how to Eat Yourself Beautiful with mouth-watering recipes that everyone will enjoy.

Many of us think that vitamins and minerals come only from vegetables, salads, and fruit and that the rest of our meals are—well, just that—the rest of our meals. But you'll learn from these recipes that the whole meal, from the first course through dessert, can provide optimum beauty potential. If using three beauty foods in a salad is good, five are even better. And you'll also learn little tricks like adding sesame seeds, which are packed with vitamin B complex and fiber, using whole-grain products wherever possible, and cutting down on fats by simmering casserole ingredients in broth instead of sautéing them.

We've listed the vitamins and minerals in specific foods at the end of each recipe to help familiarize you with where to find them. And over and over again—because you can't hear good news too often—you'll find talk of lustrous hair with lots of body, young-looking skin, chip-resistant nails and healthy teeth, and the radiance that comes from overall good health. When you eat for beauty, it's a lifelong strategy; once every three weeks won't do it.

When you start including more of these foods in your diet, you'll notice an increasing feeling of vitality and well-being after just a few days. It's just your body's way of thanking you for all the good foods you're giving it. There's lots of variety here, and as you become more familiar with these recipes you may want to try some variations of your own.

However you do it, you'll see firsthand what these beauty foods can do for you—powerful persuasions to keep you eating all these good things. No one can resist being beautiful!

Beauty Appetizers

We'll start with raw vegetables, or crudités. These do the most for your beauty potential because they contain, in their most concentrated form, all of the beauty vitamins and many of the beauty minerals as well as trace elements.

CRISP MAGIC

1/4 *head green cabbage, shredded*

1/2 *apple, chopped*

10 *walnut halves, finely chopped*

1 *small head leaf lettuce*

Wash and drain the lettuce leaves and tear them into bite-sized pieces. Combine these with the other ingredients.

BENEFIT: Crisp Magic promotes clear skin and good vision because of its high content of vitamins A, C, E, and some of the vitamin B complex, as well as calcium, potassium, and zinc.

FLOWERING ORANGE

1 *large orange, peeled and separated into sections*

1/2 *head green cabbage, shredded*

8 *almonds, chopped*

1/2 *stalk of leek, finely chopped (you can substitute two scallions if leeks aren't available)*

1 *bunch lamb's lettuce (or watercress)*

Separate the lamb's lettuce; wash and dry it thoroughly. Mix with the shredded cabbage. Put the mixture on a plate and arrange the orange sections in a circle on the bed of greens. Sprinkle with the chopped leeks and almonds.

BENEFIT: Flowering Orange contains vitamins A, C, E, and some of the vitamin B complex. It helps keep your skin young-looking and blemish free.

PINK BLUSH

S E R V E S   T W O

2 *red beets, peeled and chopped in small pieces*
1 *apple, unpeeled, thinly sliced*
$1/2$ *onion, peeled and very finely chopped*
5-6 *stalks of dill*

Arrange the apple slices on a plate. Top with the chopped beets, onion, and dill.

BENEFIT: Pink Blush contains vitamin B complex, fatty acids, and vitamins A, C, E, and K, as well as calcium and potassium. With all of these goodies, it helps to moisturize your hair and skin. Moreover, you'll have that inner glow that comes from a lot of vitamin C.

The minerals also help promote strong teeth, hair, and nails, and the fiber, which is abundant in beets, will stimulate your digestion and keep your complexion clear.

BEAUTY GREENS

2 *heads red lettuce (radicchio)*

1 *head Bibb lettuce*

1 *avocado, peeled and sliced,*
  sprinkled with juice of $1/2$ a lemon

1 *bunch of watercress*

Wash the greens, dry them thoroughly, and tear them into bite-sized pieces. Combine these with the avocado slices and toss.

BENEFIT: Beauty Greens gives you vitamins A, C, E, and K and some of the vitamin B complex. These are wonderful for glowing, blemish free skin.

Tomato Italiano

3 ripe tomatoes, thinly sliced
1/2 onion, peeled and finely chopped
1 bunch of watercress
4 ounces mozzarella or goat cheese

Slice the cheese thinly and layer the slices alternately with the tomato slices on a platter. Wash and drain the watercress leaves. Sprinkle watercress and chopped onion over the cheese and tomato.

BENEFIT: Mozzarella and goat cheese contain the essential fatty acids that are so important for vitality and for beautiful skin and hair. Tomato Italiano also has an abundance of vitamins A, C, E, and K, which increase your resistance to the effects of stress, pollution, and fatigue.

Season the Beauty Appetizers with one of the Beauty Dressings and serve them with whole-grain bread, toast, or crackers, all of which contain a lot of the vitamin B complex and fiber. Or, you can make a meal out of crudités by adding a hard-boiled egg, some cottage cheese, or mozzarella—all of which contain a wealth of vitamins and minerals.

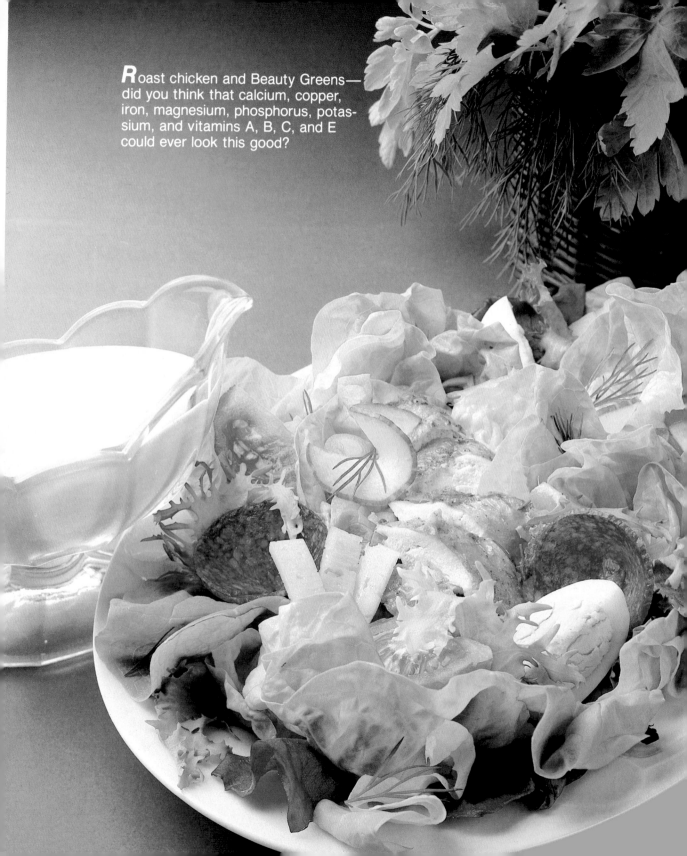

Roast chicken and Beauty Greens—did you think that calcium, copper, iron, magnesium, phosphorus, potassium, and vitamins A, B, C, and E could ever look this good?

Beauty Salads

Next are some salads that you'll enjoy with the beauty dressings in the following section.

PROTEIN PLUS

SERVES FOUR TO FIVE

4 hard-boiled eggs, sliced in circles or quartered
1 head Bibb lettuce
2 heads radicchio
1/2 head Boston lettuce
4 ounces lamb's lettuce
1 bunch of watercress
1 stalk of leek, finely chopped

Wash and thoroughly dry the greens, and tear them into bite-sized pieces. Combine and toss with the sliced eggs and chopped leeks.

BENEFIT: Protein Plus will benefit the skin, hair, teeth, eyes, and nails because the varieties of lettuce contain lots of vitamin C and smaller quantities of vitamins A, D, E, and K. The eggs provide vitamins A, B_2, D, and E in addition to sulfur (which is one of *the* beauty minerals for your skin and hair), zinc, iron, phosphorus, and several unsaturated fatty acids.

Eggs are somewhat controversial because of their high cholesterol content. But they do contain protein, one of the body's most basic building blocks, and are chockfull of vitamins and minerals. You might want to check with your doctor about how many eggs you should include in your diet.

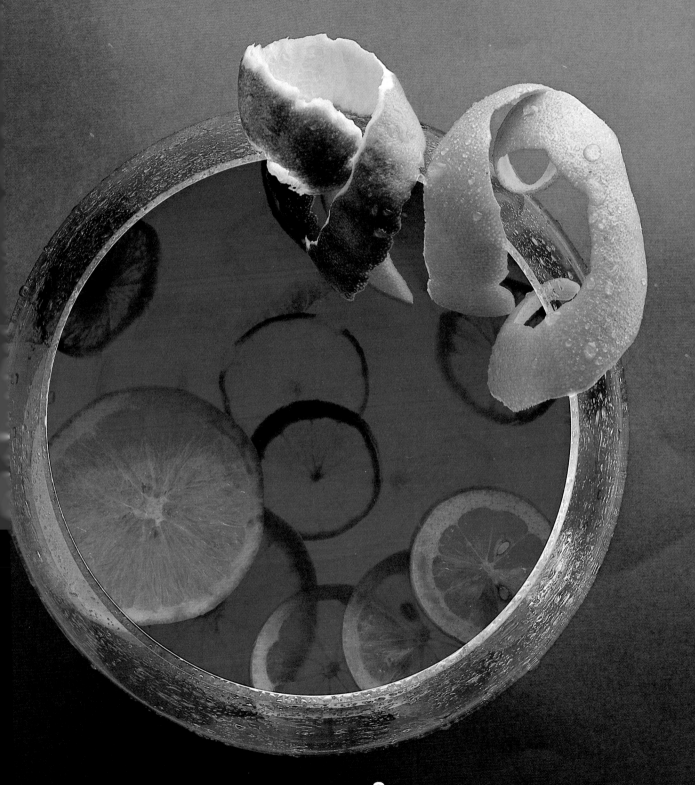

Sweet Temptations, the not-guilty desserts

SUNNY SALAD

1 *apple, coarsely chopped*

6 *carrots, scraped and shredded*

1 *head green cabbage, shredded*

4 *ounces goat cheese, cut in small pieces*

1 *ounce raisins*

2 *tablespoons mixed chopped nuts*
   (walnuts, almonds, hazelnuts, etc.)

Combine all the ingredients and toss gently.

BENEFIT: Because it contains raw vegetables, nuts, and goat cheese, the Sunny Salad contains all the vitamins we need for beauty and health. Raw carrots and cabbage have a high fiber content, which helps prevent constipation.

The carotene in carrots, which ensures even tanning (for the *limited* time that you spend in the sun), is another beauty plus. And so is the iron contained in the raisins, which counteracts fatigue.

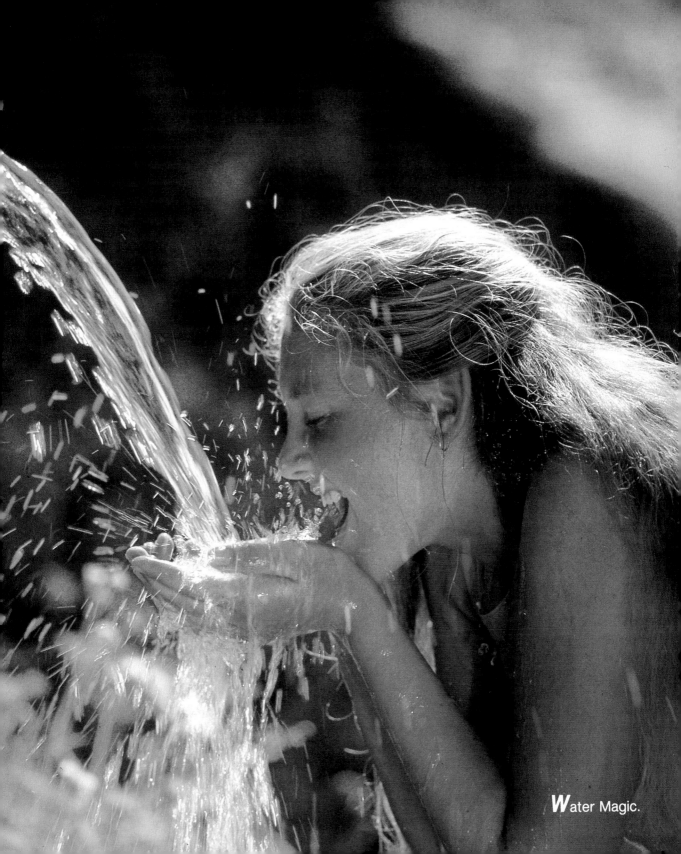

Water Magic.

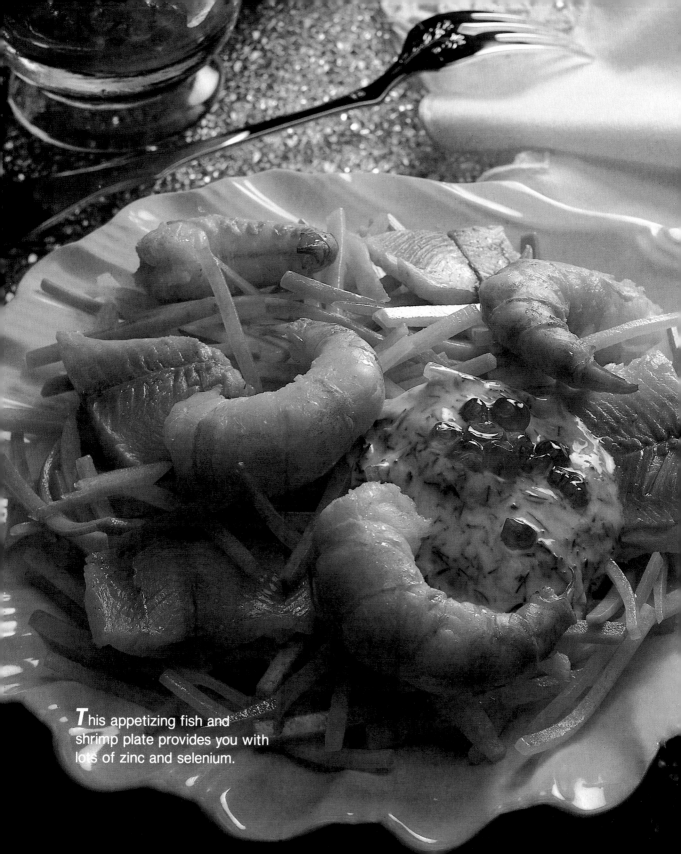

This appetizing fish and shrimp plate provides you with lots of zinc and selenium.

SUMMER SALAD

1 peach, sliced
4–5 lettuce leaves
10–12 cherries, pitted
$1/2$ cucumber, washed and thinly sliced
6 almonds, chopped

Wash and dry the lettuce leaves and spread them on a plate. Top the lettuce with peach and cucumber slices, arrange the cherries on these, and sprinkle the chopped almonds over the entire arrangement.

BENEFIT: Summer Salad has vitamin A, some of the vitamin B complex, and lots of vitamins C, E, and K.

This salad primarily helps to promote beautiful skin, although these vitamins give a lift to your entire system. The nuts also contain zinc, which is excellent for your hair.

This is one of the author's favorite snacks.

SKIN SMOOTHIE

    1 *kohlrabi, peeled and cut into thin strips*
    1 *apple, chopped*
    1 *tablespoon pumpkin seeds*
    1 *hard-boiled egg, chopped*
  ¹/₂ *head Bibb lettuce*
  ¹/₄ *green pepper, cut in thin strips*

Wash and drain the lettuce and tear it into bite-sized pieces. Combine with the remaining ingredients.

BENEFIT: As its name promises, Skin Smoothie contains everything you need for clear, young-looking skin. It provides you with vitamin A, the vitamin B complex, and vitamins C, D, E, and K. The egg and the pumpkin seeds also contain sulfur, which makes your hair lustrous and easy to handle.

HAIRGLOW

$^1/_2$ *head small Chinese cabbage*
1 *pear, chopped*
8 *walnut halves, chopped*
1 *bunch of watercress*
2 *tablespoons cottage cheese*

Wash and dry the cabbage (separating the leaves to remove sand or soil) and the watercress. Cut or tear these into bite-sized pieces, combine, and place on a plate. Top with cottage cheese in a mound and sprinkle with the chopped pear and walnuts.

BENEFIT: Hairglow contains lots of vitamin A and the vitamin B complex. Help yourself to this one often and you'll see your hair really shine. It's also great for your nails and teeth.

Beauty Dressings

Our salad dressings are also storehouses of beauty ingredients, so you're supplementing your intake of beauty aids when you use them. Most of them are easily made in a blender, and they will keep in your refrigerator for two to three days.

YOGHURT SMOOTHIE

S E R V E S   T W O

1/4 *cup plain low-fat yoghurt*
  2 *tablespoons lemon juice*
  3 *pitted apricots*
  1 *teaspoon sea salt*

Put all of the ingredients in a blender and blend at high speed until smooth.

BENEFIT: Yoghurt, without sugar or jam, is a beauty constant that contains the vitamin B complex, vitamin A, and vitamin D. Besides the vitamins, it provides good bacteria that help your intestinal tract do its job. We think that yoghurt is such an important beauty source that we're going to digress a little and give you our favorite recipe for making it. That way you can always have it on hand.

YOGHURT

MAKES TWO CUPS

$1/3$ cup plain low-fat yoghurt
2 tablespoons powdered skim milk
$1^1/2$ cups skim milk

Mix the yoghurt starter and powered and liquid skim milks thoroughly; cover and let stand in a warm place for four to six hours. Then, refrigerate the yoghurt at least three hours before using.

Now, back to the beauty dressings.

CITRUSSSSSSS

SERVES TWO

4 tablespoons lemon juice
4 tablespoons orange juice
2 tablespoons low-fat yoghurt
1 tablespoon vinegar
   herbal seasoning and pepper

Put all the ingredients in a blender and blend at high speed until smooth.

BENEFIT: The masses of vitamin C in citrus fruits give your skin that marvelous glow from within and also boost your immunity against disease.

FRENCH KISS

S E R V E S   O N E   T O   T W O

2 *tablespoons vinegar*

2 *tablespoons cold-pressed olive oil*

1 *teaspoon Dijon mustard*

2 *tablespoons low-fat milk*

herbal seasoning and pepper

Put all the ingredients in a blender and blend at high speed until smooth.

BENEFIT: Cold-pressed olive oil has lots of vitamin E, which is good for your whole body. Unfortunately, olive oil is also high in calories, so don't have too much of this dressing.

LATIN LOVING

S E R V E S   T W O

1 *ripe avocado, peeled and chopped*

3 *tablespoons lemon juice*

3 *tablespoons low-fat yoghurt*

1/2 *onion, peeled and cut up for the blender*

herbal seasoning and pepper

Put all the ingredients into a blender and blend at high speed until smooth.

BENEFIT: There are lots of vitamins A, B, C, and D in this avocado dressing. Also, avocados themselves are loaded with minerals, calcium, phosphorus, and potassium.

HAWAIIAN NIGHT

  1 *tomato, peeled, seeded, and chopped*
  1 *teaspoon tomato paste*
  1 *hard-boiled egg*
$^1/_4$ *onion, peeled and cut up for the blender*
  4 *tablespoons low-fat yoghurt*
  1 *tablespoon vinegar*
    herbal seasoning and pepper

Put all the ingredients in a blender and blend at high speed until smooth.

BENEFIT: Vitamins A, B_2, D, and E work for you in the Hawaiian Night, as do the beauty minerals sulfur, zinc, iron, and phosphorus.

HONEY LEMON

2 *tablespoons lemon juice*
1 *egg yolk*
$1/4$ *cup low-fat yoghurt*
1 *level teaspoon honey*
herbal seasoning and pepper

Put all the ingredients in the top of a double boiler, over water boiling at medium heat. Stir continuously until the dressing is thick and creamy. Serve cold.

BENEFIT: Honey Lemon provides you with B vitamins from the yoghurt, vitamin C from the lemon juice, and zinc, sulfur, and iron from the egg yolk. All of these are goodies for luxuriant hair and youthful skin.

Beauty Snacks

Keep these snacks all made up in your refrigerator, and when you've got the "nibblies," reach for them instead of something that is not so good for you. You might also serve them as a first course or as side dishes with a main course.

GUACAMOLE ROLLIES

SERVES THREE TO FOUR

12 *large lettuce leaves*
12 *toothpicks*
Filling
  1 *avocado, peeled and chopped*
  1 *tomato, chopped*
  1 *green pepper, chopped*
1/4 *onion, peeled and chopped*
  1 *thin slice of whole-grain bread*
  2 *pinches herbal seasoning*

For the filling, blend the ingredients in a blender. Make sure the mixture doesn't get too thin, because you'll want to spread it. (You can add a tiny bit more bread in case it's too thin.) Spread the filling on lettuce leaves. Roll each leaf and secure it with a toothpick.

BENEFIT: Guacamole Rollies are storehouses of vitamins, especially vitamin C, so they're marvelous for clear, glowing skin.

Lusty Tomatoes

4 tomatoes

1 onion, peeled and finely chopped

1 tablespoon mustard

3 tablespoons soybean sprouts

2 ounces goat cheese

1 tablespoon chopped parsley

Cut the top off each tomato and scoop out the insides. Turn the empty tomatoes upside down and let them drain. Mix the other ingredients with the tomato insides and stuff this mixture back into the tomato cups. Serve with toasted whole-grain bread.

BENEFIT: Lusty Tomatoes contain lots of vitamins A and C, and that means clear vision, healthy skin, and a big boost for your immune system.

Beauty Soups

These will surprise you because they are so easy to make in your blender. They taste delicious and, like all of our recipes, they are filled to the brim with beauty components. These soups are all made with raw vegetables and fruits, because that's the best way to retain all those valuable vitamins and fiber substances. If you'd like hot soup for a chilly day, heat these soups gently, but don't let them boil or you will lose the good vitamins.

APOLLO SOUP

S E R V E S   T W O

10 *large carrots, scraped and cut up for the blender*
   juice of 1/2 lemon
1/2 *onion, peeled and cut up for the blender*
 1 *green pepper, seeded and cut up for the blender*
1/4 *cup ground sunflower seeds*
 1 *cube vegetable stock dissolved in 1/4 cup hot water*
1/2 *cup plain low-fat yoghurt*
 2 *egg yolks*

Blend the first six ingredients thoroughly. Beat the egg yolks very well and mix them with the yoghurt. Stir this mixture into the soup. Garnish with chopped chives and serve chilled.

BENEFIT: Apollo Soup contains vitamins A and C and most of the vitamin B complex, as well as protein and the most important fatty acids. It's wonderful for silky, manageable hair and sparkling eyes.

GUACAMOLE GUSTO

   2 *avocados, peeled, with pits removed*
     juice and grated rind of 1 lemon
 $1/2$ *cucumber, washed*
   1 *zucchini, washed and cut up for the blender*
   1 *cup apple juice*
 $1/2$ *cube vegetable stock dissolved in $1/2$ cup hot water*
   1 *bunch lamb's lettuce*

Blend all the ingredients except one-quarter of the cucumber and a few leaves of lettuce. Garnish the soup with the cucumber, finely chopped, and with the lettuce leaves.

BENEFIT: Guacamole Gusto contains vitamins A, C, and E as well as vitamins B_1 and B_2. Help yourself to this soup for youthful, clear skin.

TOMATO CRISP

  4 tomatoes, seeded and cut into large chunks
$^1/_4$ cup yoghurt
$^1/_2$ avocado, peeled
$^1/_2$ onion, peeled and cut up for the blender
$^1/_2$ cube vegetable stock dissolved in $^1/_2$ cup hot water
 20 string beans

Blend all the ingredients except the string beans. Chop the beans finely and sprinkle them over the soup.

BENEFIT: Tomato Crisp contains primarily vitamins A and C and is marvelous for sharp vision, lustrous hair, and clear skin.

Gazpacho

1 cucumber

1 green pepper

1 onion, peeled

4 tomatoes

1 small bunch each of dill, parsley, and basil

2 tablespoons vinegar

1/4 cup plain yoghurt

herbal seasoning and pepper

1 pint tomato juice

Reserve two tomatoes and half of the cucumber and green pepper and onion; dice them.

Blend the remainder of the ingredients. Garnish with the diced vegetables and serve ice cold, accompanied by toasted whole-grain bread.

BENEFIT: Gazpacho contains lots of vitamins C, A, and some of the vitamin B complex, as well as calcium and potassium. It's especially good for soft, supple skin and beautiful, shiny hair.

CUCUMBER SHINE

   2 *cucumbers, washed and cut up for the blender*
3/4 *cup plain low-fat yoghurt*
   1 *onion, peeled and cut up for the blender*
     juice of 1/2 lemon
   1 *small bunch of dill*
   1 *level teaspoon paprika*
     herbal seasoning and pepper

Blend all the ingredients and serve very cold.

BENEFIT: Cucumber Shine contains vitamins A, B_1 and B_2, C, E, and K, as well as the beauty minerals calcium, magnesium, phosphorus, and potassium. Its effects are similar to those of Gazpacho.

TOMATO JOGGER

4 large tomatoes, peeled

1 onion, peeled and cut up for the blender

1 small bunch each of parsley and chives

1 tablespoon tomato paste

4 tablespoons yoghurt

2 tablespoons ground sunflower seeds

1 tablespoon ground sesame seeds

1 teaspoon mustard

Peel the tomatoes by plunging them into hot water, then cold. The skin will then pull off easily with a knife. Cut them up for the blender. Reserve the chives and blend all the other ingredients. Chop the chives finely and use as a garnish.

BENEFIT: The Tomato Jogger is packed with goodies. It contains vitamins A, C, E, and K as well as all the members of the vitamin B complex, together with protein and the minerals calcium, chromium, iron, magnesium, potassium, and zinc.

Ingesting all of these beauty ingredients at once boosts the entire system and results in glossy hair, healthy teeth, and an overall feeling of well-being.

GOLDMINE SOUP

$^3/_4$ *cup low-fat cottage cheese*

$^3/_4$ *cup plain low-fat yoghurt*

  1 *large bunch of watercress, washed and drained*

  1 *hard-boiled egg, coarsely chopped*

  1 *cucumber, washed and cut up for the blender*

  1 *teaspoon mustard*

    herbal seasoning and pepper

  8 *walnut halves, ground*

Reserve a little of the watercress for a garnish and blend all the other ingredients. This soup can be served cold or warm, but it should never boil.

BENEFIT: We've christened it Goldmine Soup because that's what it is—a goldmine of beauty vitamins and minerals. It contains vitamin A, all of the B vitamins, which are so important for our overall vitality and our immune system, and also vitamins C, D, and E. In addition, it provides the beauty minerals calcium, iron, magnesium, phosphorus, potassium, selenium, and sulfur. Radiant, youthful skin that's perfectly balanced, lustrous hair, and strong nails will be yours when you include this soup in your diet.

FROM NUTS TO SOUP

$^2/_3$ *cup chopped walnuts*

 1 *small onion, peeled and cut up for the blender*

 2 *cubes vegetable stock dissolved in 2 cups water*

 1 *large bunch of watercress*

 1 *stalk of leek*

$^1/_3$ *cup plain low-fat yoghurt*

   herbal seasoning and pepper

Reserve a few watercress leaves for a garnish and blend the rest of the ingredients. This soup can be served cold or warm, with the watercress floating prettily on top. From Nuts to Soup is especially good with toasted whole-grain bread and a green salad.

BENEFIT: The nuts in the soup give you quite a lot of protein and the three most important unsaturated fatty acids. A deficiency in these acids causes all kinds of skin problems, including dandruff. So help yourself to this soup and keep your skin dewy and youthful.

Water Magic

You've got to have water and lots of it. Water is essential for blemish free skin and a beautiful, healthy body. It helps your digestion, flushes your kidneys, and prevents constipation.

Now, you don't have to worry about force-feeding yourself the famous six to eight glasses a day. That quantity refers to your total fluid intake, which can include herb teas, freshly prepared fruit and vegetable juices, decaffeinated coffee substitutes, low-fat milk, and buttermilk. You should stay away from whole milk, strong coffee, and sugared sodas. But, getting back to water for a second, it's probably the best thirst quencher there is. Get yourself a pretty crystal glass and make sipping mineral or tap water a treat, knowing that at the same time you're doing wonderful things for yourself.

Beauty Drinks

These beauty drinks provide a great way to take in lots of fluid. These magic potions made from fresh fruits and vegetables have been served at elegant health spas for years. They revitalize your system, because fresh uncooked fruits and vegetables consist solely of beauty ingredients. They provide vitamins and minerals, fiber, lots of water, and enzymes, all of which give you a great feeling of physical well-being.

You'll see and feel a difference if you concentrate on these beauty drinks and salads for a few days. (But make sure you talk with your doctor before you make any change in your diet.) You'll feel peppier and look better. Your skin will look youthful, your hair will gleam, and your eyes will sparkle.

Try to drink all of the beauty drinks when they're fresh, because they lose their beauty effect when they're refrigerated for more than one day.

LIQUID GOLD

S E R V E S T W O

5 carrots, scraped and prepared for the blender
1/2 apple, peeled and seeded
1/2 cucumber
1 orange, peeled and divided into sections
  low-sodium salt and pepper
1 level teaspoon honey

Put all the ingredients into a blender and liquefy.

BENEFIT: Liquid Gold contains vitamin A, some of the vitamin B complex, and vitamins C, D, E, and K. It's great for digestion and for youthful, blemish free skin (as well as carotene to help your *careful* tanning).

CUCUMBER COOLER

S E R V E S T W O

1 cucumber, washed and cut up for the blender
1 small bunch of dill
  juice of 1/2 lemon
1 cup buttermilk
1/4 cube vegetable stock dissolved in 2 tablespoons of water

Put all ingredients in a blender and liquefy.

BENEFIT: Cucumber Cooler is marvelous for hair and skin. It contains vitamins A and C and some of the vitamin B complex, as well as the beauty minerals calcium and phosphorus.

SUMMER BOUNTY

1 *peach, pitted and cut up for the blender*
2 *apricots, pitted and cut up for the blender*
1 *orange, peeled and sectioned*
$1/2$ *head leaf lettuce, washed and dried*
$1/4$ *cup low-fat yoghurt*

Liquefy all the ingredients and garnish the drink with mint leaves and grapes.

BENEFIT: Summer Bounty contains lots and lots of vitamin C, as well as the beauty minerals iron and magnesium. It tastes absolutely delicious, it's wonderful for your skin, and if you're feeling a little tired, it gives you more pep and helps to fortify your immune system.

TOMATO CREAM

4 tomatoes, peeled (as described for Tomato Jogger)
1 avocado, peeled and with the pit removed
  juice of 1 lemon
$1/4$ cup buttermilk
$1/2$ apple, seeded and cut up for the blender
  one pinch each of herbal seasoning and pepper
1 small bunch of parsley

Put all the ingredients in a blender and liquefy.

BENEFIT: Tomato Cream contains vitamins A and C, as well as the beauty minerals potassium, calcium, and magnesium. It promotes lustrous hair and good vision.

CHERRY COCO

about 20 cherries, pitted
1 tablespoon shredded coconut
2 oranges, peeled and sectioned
4 apricots, pitted and cut in pieces
2 tablespoons water

Put all the ingredients in a blender and liquefy.

BENEFIT: Lots of vitamin C, some of the vitamin B complex, as well as calcium, magnesium, and zinc make Cherry Coco great for hair, skin, and nails.

PEACH 'N APPLE SODA

  1 *peach, pitted and cut up*
  1 *apple, seeded and cut up*
  4 *ounces soda water*
  4 *ounces buttermilk*
10 *seedless grapes*
  1 *small bunch of dill, washed and drained*
  6 *chopped almonds*

Put all the ingredients into a blender, liquefy, and garnish with dill sprigs and grapes.

BENEFIT: Peach 'n Apple Soda has a fresh, sparkling taste. It contains many of the B vitamins as well as vitamins A, C, E, and K, and the beauty minerals calcium, manganese, and potassium. It's good for beautiful, supple skin all over your body.

BLACK BEAUTY

$^1/_8$ *cup club soda or mineral water*

$^1/_2$ *pint blueberries*

$^1/_4$ *cup currant juice*

$^1/_2$ *cup buttermilk*

  3 *tablespoons yoghurt*

Put all the ingredients in a blender and liquefy.

BENEFIT: Black Beauty contains masses of vitamins C, A, and D and the minerals calcium and potassium. It promotes younger looking skin, and the vitamin C also helps you avoid colds and other infections.

PINEAPPLE ZOOM

$1/2$ *cup club soda or mineral water*
$1/2$ *pineapple, peeled and cut into chunks*
$1/4$ *cup buttermilk*
  3 *tablespoons low-fat yoghurt*
  1 *level tablespoon honey*

Put all the ingredients in a blender and liquefy. Garnish with 1 tablespoon of sesame seeds.

BENEFIT: Pineapple Zoom contains vitamins A, C, D, and K as well as vitamins B_1 and B_2. In addition, it provides the beauty minerals calcium, phosphorus, and potassium. This combination will clear your skin and make your hair gleam.

We might suggest sesame seeds as a garnish for all sorts of dishes. They're an easy way to add a highly packed beauty supplement to your food. Sesame seeds contain vitamins B, E, and F in abundant quantities and they also have calcium, copper, chromium, iron, manganese, potassium, and zinc, as well as lots of fiber. This combination of vitamins and minerals is especially important for your skin. Vitamin F also prevents arteriosclerosis because it helps the body to rid itself of excess cholesterol.

Beauty Entrées

Protein is very important for youthful, clear skin, and luxuriant hair; and it's essential for all of the growth and regeneration processes. High-protein foods like fish, eggs, and lean meats contain many of the beauty minerals, particularly sulfur, potassium, phosphorus, zinc, and iron. In this section you will find delicious recipes for all the protein sources.

Soufflés

One of our favorite ways to obtain protein is soufflés. They're quick and easy to prepare and they appeal to our modern desire for light food. Here are two delicious soufflés that you can serve for lunch or dinner. Accompany them with some good whole-grain bread and Beauty Greens, or any other salad that appeals to you, and you have a nutritious, light meal. You'll enjoy the food and you'll feel good thinking about all the beauty benefits you're getting.

MUSHROOM SOUFFLÉ

1 *tablespoon butter*

2 *tablespoons whole-wheat flour*

1 *cup hot low-fat milk*

2 *tablespoons grated Parmesan cheese*

1 *pinch nutmeg*

4 *egg yolks, beaten*

5 *egg whites, at room temperature*

1/2 *pound mushrooms, thinly sliced*

2 *tablespoons olive oil*

2 *small onions, finely chopped*
   herbal seasoning and pepper

Butter a one-quart soufflé dish and preheat the oven to 400°.

Make a white sauce by melting the butter over high heat and sautéing the flour in the melted butter, taking care not to let the mixture turn brown. Add the hot milk and stir continuously until the sauce thickens. When the sauce has thickened, turn the heat off and stir in the Parmesan cheese, nutmeg, herbal seasoning, and pepper. Set the sauce aside.

Over medium heat, sauté the onions in the olive oil until they're golden and limp and then add the sliced mushrooms. Let the mixture sauté just until the mushrooms have turned color. Add the mushroom-onion mixture to the white sauce. Next, add the egg yolks as follows: Stir 5-6 tablespoons of the hot sauce into the dish with the beaten yolks, then add this mixture to the rest of the sauce. (Otherwise, you'll be making scrambled eggs when the yolks suddenly come in contact with the hot sauce.) Beat the egg whites and add them to the rest in three portions, *stirring* in the first portion and *folding* in the other two. Bake for approximately forty minutes until the soufflé is high and puffy. Serve immediately.

CRAB SOUFFLÉ

- 2 tablespoons butter
- 3 tablespoons whole-wheat flour
- 1 cup hot low-fat milk
- 8 tablespoons grated Parmesan cheese
- 1/2 pound cooked crabmeat, thoroughly drained and flaked
- 4 egg yolks, beaten
- 5 egg whites, at room temperature
  herbal seasoning and pepper
- 1 large bunch of chives

Butter a one-quart soufflé dish and preheat the oven to 400°.

Make a white sauce by melting the butter over high heat and sautéing the flour in the melted butter, taking care not to let the mixture turn brown. Add the hot milk and stir continuously until the sauce thickens. When the sauce has thickened, turn the heat off and stir in the Parmesan cheese, crabmeat, chives, herbal seasoning, and pepper. Add the egg yolks as follows: Stir 5-6 tablespoons of the hot crab mixture into the dish with the beaten yolks, then add the mixture to the rest of the sauce. Beat the egg whites and add them to the rest in three portions, *stirring* in the first portion and carefully *folding* in the other two. Bake for forty-five to fifty minutes until the soufflé is high and puffy.

BENEFIT: These soufflés contain the beauty minerals zinc, sulfur, iron, and phosphorus, as well as unsaturated fatty acids and vitamins A, B$_2$, D, and E. Zinc is very important for healthy hair, and it also works with vitamin C, sulfur, and potassium to make your skin less susceptible to blemishes.

Fish and Seafood

Fish and seafood are very special beauty foods. Many kinds of fish and seafood contain very little fat. But we're also beginning to learn that even those that are considered to be fatty fish, such as salmon, tuna, and the crab and shrimp once feared for their cholesterol, are very good for you.

It seems that the fatty fish and high-cholesterol seafoods are rich in unsaturated fats known as omega-3 fatty acids. These have been found to be lower in cholesterol and triglycerides, as shown in a recent study at the Oregon Health Sciences University in Portland. Dr. William Connor, professor of medicine and head of the clinical nutrition department, worked with healthy volunteers and patients who had very high blood fats and gave them a pound of salmon daily. Blood fats dropped and, according to Dr. Connor, "the higher the blood fats were to begin with, the greater the fall."

In addition, fish and seafood contain high levels of the minerals iodine, calcium, sodium, zinc, iron, phosphorus, potassium, and sulfur—almost all of the beauty minerals.

Below are a few delicious and easy fish recipes. You can try all kinds of fish and seafood, just don't prepare them with too much in the way of fats or caloric mayonnaise.

YOUTH DEW TROUT

4 *trouts (without heads), split and boned*
   about 4 tablespoons seasoned whole-wheat flour
$1/4$ *cup slivered almonds*
   low-sodium salt and pepper
1 *bunch of dill*
1 *lemon, cut in slices*
1 *tablespoon sunflower oil*

Stuff the trout with the lemon slices and dill, roll them in the flour, and season them with salt and pepper. Spread oil on both sides and sprinkle slivered almonds on top. Broil for approximately eight minutes, turning the fish once.

Baked potatoes (which contain some protein, lots of fiber, and a few of the B vitamins) and a mixed green salad go very nicely with the trout.

BENEFIT: Youth Dew Trout contains lots of iodine, which promotes glistening hair and moisturizes skin against dryness and wrinkles. In addition, there are the vitamins B_2 and B_6, niacin, biotin, and the minerals copper, iron, manganese, potassium, sulfur, and zinc.

The almonds also have vitamin E and a number of unsaturated fatty acids that are necessary for glowing, blemish free skin.

Youth Dew Trout is a real winner, or rather, you're the winner when you eat it. It's good for your skin and hair and supplies your body with all the minerals you need to feel good.

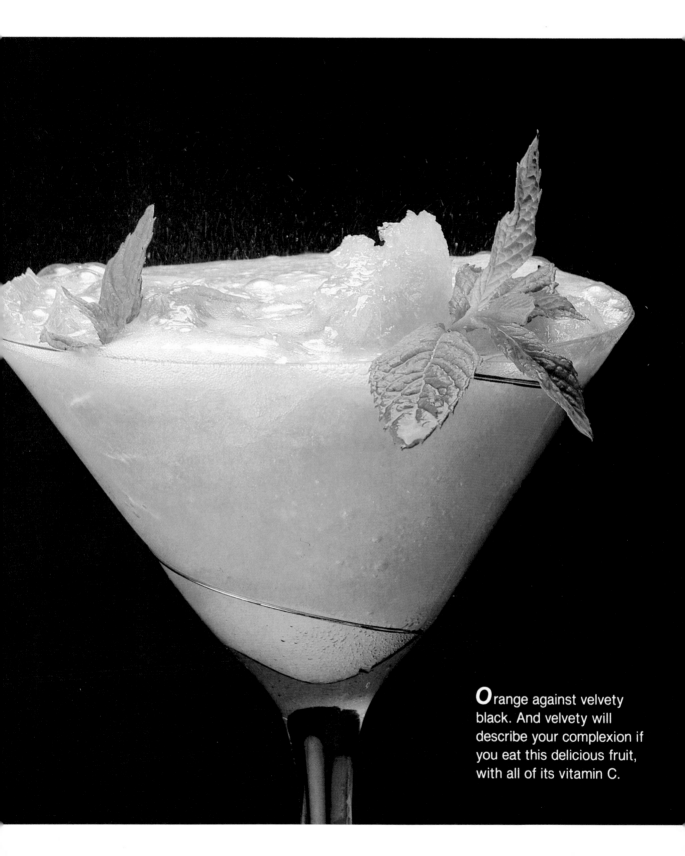

Orange against velvety black. And velvety will describe your complexion if you eat this delicious fruit, with all of its vitamin C.

TURBOT CHIVES ALIVE

4 *turbot filets*
1 *tablespoon olive oil*
   herbal seasoning and pepper
   juice of 1/2 *lemon*
3/4 *cup plain low-fat yoghurt*
4 *tablespoons chopped chives*

Spread oil on both sides of the filets and season them with the herbal seasoning, pepper, and lemon juice. Broil them for about ten minutes, turning the filets once. Put them on a hot platter and place it in a previously warmed oven with the heat turned off.

Mix the yoghurt with the chives and some of the herbal seasoning and pepper, and heat this mixture very gently. Pour the chive sauce over the broiled fish and serve immediately. Turbot Chives Alive are good with wild rice and a tossed green salad.

BENEFIT: These filets provide the beauty minerals copper, iodine, potassium, sulfur, and zinc, as well as several of the B vitamins and a little vitamin C in the chives. All of these contribute to a healthy nervous system and increased vigor. The sulfur, in particular, does wonders for your hair and skin.

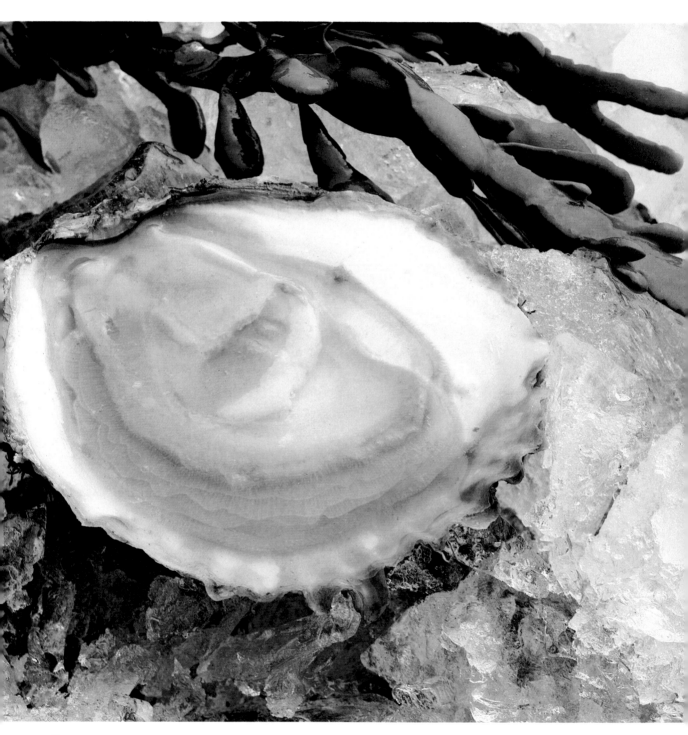

*L*ook at this oyster and imagine glossy hair. That's what you'll get from the iodine in seafood.

FLOUNDER ITALIANA

- 6 *flounder filets*
- 3 *tomatoes, sliced*
- 2 *lemons, sliced*
- 3 *pitted black olives, chopped*
- 1 *tablespoon chopped fresh or dried basil*
- 2 *onions, peeled and cut in slices*
- 1 *heaping tablespoon tomato paste, dissolved in 1/4 cup vegetable stock*
- 2 *tablespoons olive oil*

Preheat the over to 350°. Grease a baking sheet with 2 teaspoons of the olive oil and reserve the rest. Place the filets on the baking sheet and sprinkle them with a little pepper. Cover the fish filets with layers of onion, tomato, and lemon slices. Pour the tomato mixture over the filets, sprinkle them with the chopped olives and basil, and drizzle them with the remaining olive oil. Bake for approximately twenty minutes.

BENEFIT: This very Mediterranean fish dish features iron, magnesium, potassium, and sulfur, minerals that contribute to glowing skin and luxuriant hair.

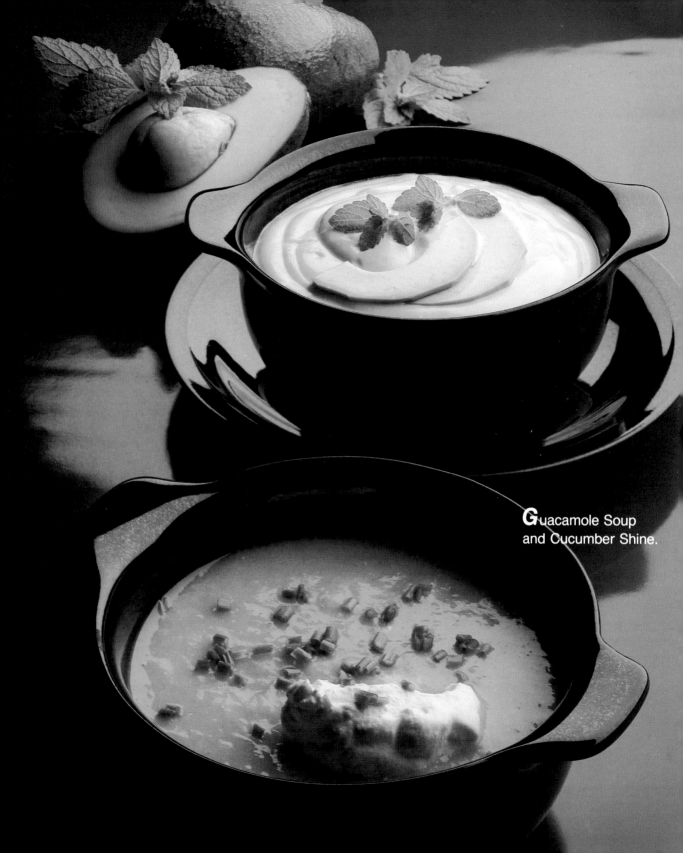

Guacamole Soup
and Cucumber Shine.

Just looking at this salad makes you feel peppy.

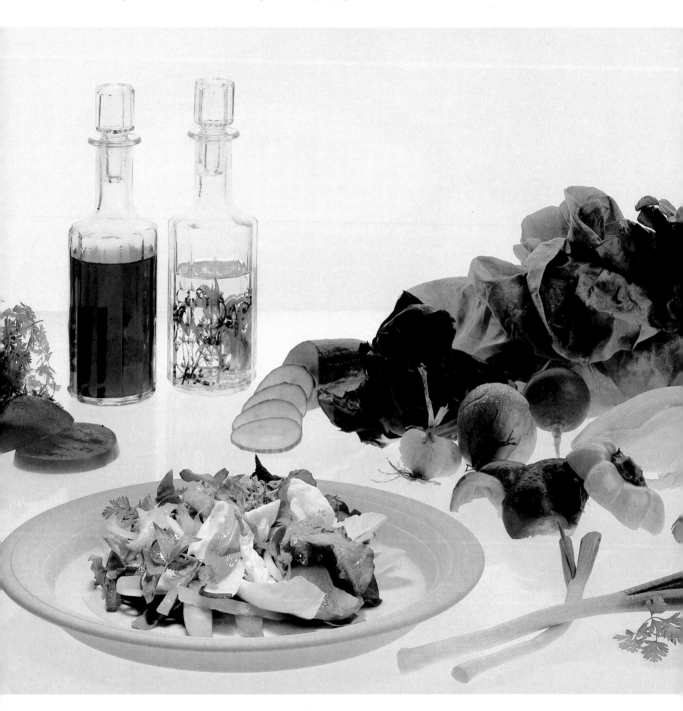

SALMON SPECTACLE

1 whole salmon, approximately 8 pounds (eviscerated)
1 quart vegetable stock
1 bunch of leeks, washed and chopped
For the garnish:
1 cucumber, very thinly sliced
  about 20 boiled shrimp
2 heads leaf lettuce, washed and drained
2 lemons, sliced
1 large bunch of parsley, washed and drained

Place the salmon, vegetable stock, and chopped leeks in a fish cooker or large covered pan; bring them to a boil slowly. Cook for three minutes, then remove the pan from the heat. Transfer the fish and stock to a large container, cover, and refrigerate.

The next day, carefully lift the cold fish out of the stock and onto a wooden board. Remove the skin. Place on a serving platter lined with the lettuce leaves. Cover the whole fish with the thinly sliced cucumbers and garnish it with the shrimp, lemon slices, and sprigs of parsley. Serve with small, whole, unpeeled boiled potatoes and dill sauce.

BENEFIT: There are so many good things for you in the Salmon Spectacle: vitamins A, B_2, B_6, B_{12}; niacin and biotin; vitamins D and K; some unsaturated fatty acids; and the minerals copper, iodine, iron, sulfur, and zinc. Sharp vision and silky hair will be your benefits here.

This is wonderful if you're entertaining a lot of people.

SHRIMPLY FINE

$^1/_2$ *pound shrimp, peeled and cooked*
$^1/_2$ *cucumber, washed and cut in thin slices*
  1 *head Bibb lettuce, washed and drained*
  2 *ounces lamb's lettuce, washed and drained*
    juice of 1 lemon
$^1/_4$ *cup Hawaiian Night*

Line a salad bowl with the lettuce leaves and arrange the cucumber slices and lamb's lettuce over them. Mix the shrimp with the lemon juice and spoon the mixture over the bed of vegetables. Top with Hawaiian Night and serve with toasted whole-grain bread.

BENEFIT: The Shrimply Fine contains vitamins A, C, and E, and some of the vitamin B complex, as well as the minerals calcium, iodine, iron, magnesium, potassium, and zinc. It's very good for maintaining youthful, elastic skin and gives a special luster to your hair.

STEAMLINED SHRIMP

S E R V E S   F O U R

1 *pound large shrimp, shelled*
3 *tablespoons corn flour*
2 *onions, peeled and thinly sliced*
4 *tomatoes, sliced*
1 *stalk of leek, sliced*
4 *tablespoons dry white wine*
2 *tablespoons soy sauce*
  pepper

Roll the shrimp in the corn flour and combine them with the vegetables. Mix the wine and soy sauce and add to the above mixture. Place the shrimp in the basket of a steamer, cover, and steam over rapidly boiling water for about five minutes. Serve on a bed of brown rice and accompany with a tomato salad.

BENEFIT: Steamlined Shrimp are a good source of iodine, selenium, and zinc. These minerals will give your hair lots of body and keep your skin youthful. Iodine is also essential for proper thyroid function.

Meat and Poultry

Eating for beauty means a well-rounded diet, one that provides you with many different nutrients from many different sources, including protein from various types of meat and poultry.

All of the meat you eat should be lean, with as much of the fat trimmed off as possible, or, in the case of poultry, with skin removed. In general, it's best to keep meat portions on the small side and to favor poultry over other meats. Beef should probably be at the bottom of our list.

B-complex vitamins occur in varying proportions in different meats, as do various minerals. So the best thing is to have a little of everything: veal, lamb, pork, beef, chicken, turkey, and, if possible, some liver. Although it causes many of us to wrinkle up our noses, liver is full of good things: lots of vitamin B, some vitamin A and iron, copper, and selenium. Well, you *can* always eat paté.

PEACHY CHICKEN SALAD

- 1/4 *chicken, roasted, skin removed*
- 1 *head leaf lettuce, washed and thoroughly dried*
- 1/2 *cucumber*
- 1 *peach, sliced and sprinkled with a little lemon juice so that it won't turn brown*
- 1 *cup cooked broccoli*
- 1/4 *cup walnut pieces*
- 1/2 *stalk of leek, very finely chopped*

Cover a serving plate with lettuce leaves and make an attractive arrangement of the cucumbers, peaches, broccoli, and nuts. Slice the chicken and put the slices on top of the other ingredients. Drizzle with vinaigrette. Serve with whole-grain bread.

BENEFIT: Peachy Chicken Salad contains vitamins A, B, C, and E and the minerals calcium, copper, iron, magnesium, manganese, phosphorus, potassium, selenium, and zinc. It combines the protein and minerals in the chicken with the vitamins and fiber in the salad ingredients, making it wonderful for our skin, hair, and nails.

TURKEY KEBABS

$^3/_4$ pound lean, uncooked turkey meat, cut in cubes
8 cherry tomatoes
2 onions, peeled and cut in chunks
1 green pepper, washed and cut in squares
8 small mushrooms
4 broiling skewers
  basting liquid (see recipe below)

Arrange the ingredients attractively on four skewers, brush them all over with the basting liquid, and broil them for about eight minutes. Turn the skewers frequently and continue basting with the liquid. If you have a pan just wide enough so that you can hang the skewers across it, they'll be easier to turn. Make sure to wear your oven mitts!

Basting liquid:
4 tablespoons olive oil
  juice of $^1/_2$ lemon
1 teaspoon mustard
$^1/_4$ cup vegetable stock
  freshly ground black pepper
2 tablespoons chopped parsley

Mix all the ingredients and brush the mixture on the turkey and vegetables. Serve the turkey kebabs with brown rice and a mixed green salad.

BENEFIT: This turkey recipe is full of protein and the minerals chromium, iodine, phosphorus, potassium, selenium, sulfur, and zinc. It is a wonderful dish for giving you beautiful coloring and lustrous hair.

BETTER BEEF BOURGUIGNON

- 2 *pounds lean beef, cut in cubes*
- 6 *tablespoons whole-wheat flour*
- 4 *tablespoons olive oil*
- 1 *tablespoon butter*
  herbal seasoning and pepper
- 2 *carrots, scraped and sliced*
- 2 *stalks of leek, sliced*
- 2 *onions, peeled and chopped*
- 1/2 *bottle red wine*
- 1/2 *cup concentrated vegetable stock*
- 6-8 *ounces small mushrooms (sliced or left whole, depending on size)*
- 1 *bunch of parsley, washed and chopped*

Preheat the oven to 350°. Coat the meat cubes with three tablespoons of flour, reserving the rest. Heat the butter and olive oil in a heavy frying pan until they're sizzling; brown the meat. Transfer the meat to a large casserole. Add four tablespoons of the red wine to the frying pan and season with the herbal seasoning and pepper. Let simmer for two minutes.

Braise the carrots, onions, and leeks in the frying pan liquid for five minutes, season, and add this mixture to the meat in the casserole.

Add the remainder of the red wine and 1/2 cup of concentrated vegetable stock to the casserole and bake in the oven for two and a half hours, or until the meat is done. Add the mushrooms fifteen minutes before the end of the cooking period.

Take a few tablespoons of gravy out of the casserole and mix them with three tablespoons of flour to make a smooth paste. Add this to the casserole to thicken the gravy. To serve, garnish with lots of chopped parsley.

BENEFIT: Better Beef Bourguignon contains lots of protein, as well as phosphorus, potassium, sulfur, and zinc. The sulfur, in particular, makes your skin glow and makes your hair fuller.

COOL BEEF SALAD

SERVES FOUR

1 pound cold, cooked lean beef

2 hard-boiled eggs

2 heads radicchio

1 head leaf lettuce

2 tomatoes

4 ounces lamb's lettuce

1 tablespoon safflower oil

1 bunch of chives

Wash and dry the lettuce leaves and slice the tomatoes. Cut the meat into thin strips and quarter the eggs.

Put the greens, tomatoes, and beef into a salad bowl and toss with vinaigrette to which the safflower oil has been added. Arrange the eggs on top, garnish with chopped chives, and sprinkle a little black pepper on the salad.

BENEFIT: This salad, which might be called a protein salad, is full of vitamins, minerals, unsaturated fatty acids, and, of course, protein. It contains vitamins A, B, C, D, E, F, and K, as well as calcium, chromium, iron, manganese, phosphorus, potassium, selenium, sulfur, and zinc. Whether you want clear, healthy skin, strong and chip-resistant nails, or an overall feeling of well-being, this salad delivers it all.

Beauty Grains

Yes, you *can* eat carbohydrates! Forget the bread, pasta, and rice myths—the ones that say you mustn't eat bread, pasta, and rice because they'll make you fat, water retentive, and generally turn you into a doughy lump. That happens only if you choose the wrong carbohydrates, the ones that are full of sugar and refined white flour. But what we have in mind are the whole-grain carbohydrates that are full of vitamin B complex and fiber. They're what we call slow-burning carbohydrates and they do just that. They're digested slowly, which keeps your energy level on an even course, with none of the dips and swings that you get with highly refined products or those that contain sugar. Once you've finished digesting the part that is digestible, the fiber goes on to rev up the rest of your digestive system. That helps prevent constipation, and we've already told you how good that is for your health and your looks. We're going to give you some delicious brown rice and pasta recipes. But you'll want to find other ways to include whole-grain products in your diet as well. Think interesting breads, think whole-wheat crackers, think oatmeal and millet and couscous. Try the Beauty Muesli that starts this section as a starter for your day.

BEAUTY MUESLI

2 tablespoons sesame seeds

2 tablespoons linseed

2 tablespoons bran

1 tablespoon oats

1 tablespoon pumpkin seeds

1/4 apple

1/4 orange

1/4 banana

1 tablespoon raisins

1 tablespoon mixed ground nuts

You can save a lot of time by making up a large amount of the dry ingredients, without the fresh fruit, at the beginning of each week. Then you can just add the fresh fruit each morning. Mix the muesli with yoghurt, milk, or buttermilk and sweeten it with a little honey.

BENEFIT: The sesame seeds contain magnesium, potassium, and calcium, and the pumpkin seeds are bursting with vitamin B complex, phosphorus, iron, and zinc. This combination of ingredients contains all the vitamins and minerals necessary for beauty, and the fiber ensures regularity. This is a great way to start the day.

RAVISHING RISOTTO

$^1/_2$ *cup brown rice*

  1 *cup vegetable stock*

  1 *tablespoon olive oil*

  1 *finely chopped onion*

  1 *cup cooked, peeled shrimp*

  1 *zucchini, washed but not peeled, thinly sliced*

  2 *tablespoons chopped basil*

In a heavy two-quart casserole, sauté the onions in the olive oil until they're golden, stir in the rice, add the vegetable stock, and immediately put on the lid. Cook over medium heat for thirty minutes.

In the meantime, braise the shrimp with the zucchini in a little vegetable stock. When the rice has finished cooking, add the shrimp, zucchini, and basil to the pot and toss lightly. Serve with a mixed salad.

BENEFIT: Ravishing Risotto contains lots of vitamin B complex, vitamin E, protein, and the beauty minerals calcium, copper, chromium, iron, iodine, magnesium, manganese, potassium, selenium, sulfur, and zinc.

This plethora of minerals and protein is a great beauty booster. Risotto Italiano is wonderful for your complexion and for gleaming hair. Because brown rice releases an even flow of calories, this dish also improves your stamina.

Although we call this risotto, the cooking procedure here is faster than the classic Italian method.

HOT RICE SALAD

$^1/_2$ *cup brown rice*

1 *cup vegetable stock*

1 *stalk of leek, finely chopped*

3 *tomatoes, washed and sliced*

$^1/_2$ *green pepper, washed and diced*

$^1/_2$ *pound goat cheese or mozzarella, cubed*

6 *pitted black olives, chopped*

2 *tablespoons olive oil*

2 *tablespoons fresh parsley, chopped*
   herbal seasoning and pepper

In a one-quart saucepan, bring the rice and stock to a boil, cover, and cook for thirty minutes. In the meantime, heat the olive oil and gently sauté the other ingredients, seasoning them with the pepper and herbal seasoning. Combine this mixture with the cooked rice and serve with a tossed salad.

BENEFIT: Hot Rice Salad contains lots of vitamin B complex and vitamins C and K, as well as calcium, chromium, iron, magnesium, manganese, phosphorus, potassium, and zinc. It gives your skin elasticity and a youthful glow, and it strengthens your nails and your immune system.

SLENDER TUNA SPAGHETTI

1 pound whole-grain spaghetti

1 garlic clove

2 tablespoons olive oil

8 tablespoons tomato paste dissolved in 1 cup water

3/4 cup flaked tuna

3 anchovies, finely chopped

herbal seasoning and pepper

2 tablespoons fresh parsley, chopped

Peel the garlic clove, mash it with the side of a knife, and sauté it briefly in olive oil. Don't let it burn. Remove the clove and discard. Add the tomato paste dissolved in water and season the sauce with herbal seasoning and pepper. Simmer for thirty minutes. Add the tuna fish and anchovies and simmer for another fifteen minutes.

Cook the spaghetti to the *al dente* stage in a large pot of boiling salted water. Mix the pasta with the sauce and chopped parsley.

BENEFIT: Slender Tuna Spaghetti provides the vitamins A, B, D, and E and the minerals calcium, copper, chromium, iodine, iron, magnesium, manganese, phosphorus, potassium, selenium, sulfur, and zinc. All of these minerals and vitamins make Slender Tuna Spaghetti a great hair and skin beautifier.

Elegant Eggplant Lasagne

  1 *pound whole-grain lasagne*

  4 *medium eggplants, sliced*

  4 *large tomatoes, sliced*

  2 *large onions, peeled and sliced*

  6 *tablespoons grated Parmesan cheese*

$1/2$ *cup plain low-fat yoghurt*

  4 *tablespoons tomato paste*

$1/4$ *cup vegetable stock*

    black pepper

Preheat the over to 350° and lightly grease a large, shallow baking dish or lasagne pan.

Salt the eggplant slices, place them in a colander, weight them down with a wooden board or whatever is handy, and let them stand for thirty minutes. This will drain out the liquid that's responsible for the bitter taste that eggplant sometimes has. Rinse the slices thoroughly, pat them dry, then sauté them very quickly in olive oil. (The trick is to put them down, turn them over, and get them out before they soak up all of the olive oil.)

Mix the tomato paste with the yoghurt and vegetable stock.

While you're working with the eggplant, cook the lasagne in a large pot of boiling water until it is *al dente,* then drain.

Alternate layers of the cooked lasagne and the eggplant slices and onion and tomato (combine the vegetables in one layer), put a little sauce and Parmesan between each layer, and put all of the remaining Parmesan on the top layer. Bake for forty to forty-five minutes.

BENEFIT: Elegant Eggplant Lasagne contains the vitamins A, B, E, and K and the beauty minerals calcium, copper, chromium, iron, manganese, phosphorus, potassium, selenium, and zinc, as well as some protein and plant fiber. This lasagne strengthens your hair and nails and promotes good eyesight.

This recipe will be popular even with guests who haven't yet discovered how to eat for beauty.

Beauty Vegetables

Whether you serve them warm or cold, cooked vegetables are another part of your lifelong beauty strategy. It's true that raw vegetables have the highest vitamin, mineral, and fiber contents. But steamed or briefly cooked vegetables that are still crisp and colorful are not far behind their raw counterparts in delivering beauty essentials. They retain lots of the good components as well as their taste. You might even begin to like vegetables that you thought you disliked because you'll really be tasting them for the first time.

A vegetable steamer might be a nice beauty investment, but you can also steam vegetables by putting them into a colander that will stand in your spaghetti pot and placing water in the bottom of the pot. Adding some herbs or spices to the water gives the vegetables a nice, subtle taste.

There are so many ways to make and serve fresh vegetables and, unless you drown them in oil or butter, they can't be bad for you. Vegetables are full of beauty vitamins and minerals, fiber, and even a little protein. We're going to present some vegetable combination recipes that give you lots of benefits and that are also nice to serve when you have guests.

SULTRY SPINACH WITH ALMONDS

$1^1/_2$ *pounds spinach, briefly steamed*

1 *large onion, peeled and chopped*

2 *cloves garlic, peeled and finely mashed*

1 *pound raw potatoes, cut in thin slices (keep these in cold water until you're ready to use them or they'll turn brown)*

2 *bay leaves*

1 *tablespoon thyme*

  grated rind of 1 lemon

  herbal seasoning and pepper

$^1/_4$ *cup slivered almonds*

4 *tablespoons olive oil*

Preheat the oven to 300°. Sauté the onions and garlic until the onion is transparent. Add the thinly sliced potatoes and cook for a few minutes. Then combine the potatoes with the spinach in a lightly greased casserole. Season with thyme, pepper, and herbal seasoning. Add about $^1/_2$ cup boiling water and stir in the lemon rind. Put the bay leaves on top and bake for forty-five minutes. Toast the slivered almonds in the oven and sprinkle them over the spinach when it's finished. Remove the bay leaves before serving.

BENEFIT: Sultry Spinach with Almonds contains vitamins A, E, F, and lots of vitamin B and the minerals calcium, chromium, iron, magnesium, manganese, and zinc. It is excellent for smooth, young-looking skin, and the unsaturated fatty acids (vitamin F) keep your hair silky.

EGGPLANT ENTIRE

  4 *medium eggplants*

  2 *large onions, peeled and chopped*

10 *tomatoes*

  3 *tablespoons parsley*

    herbal seasoning and pepper

  1 *tablespoon basil*

  1 *clove garlic*

  4 *tablespoons olive oil*

$^1/_2$ *pound mozzarella*

Preheat the oven to 325°.

Slice the eggplants in half lengthwise, take out the insides, and salt both the shells and the inside that you've chopped up. After thirty minutes, rinse the shells and insides and drain them on paper towels. Briefly sauté the shells in olive oil. Put these into a baking dish that will hold the eight shells side by side.

In the same olive oil that you used for the shells, sauté the chopped onions until they're transparent, then add six of the tomatoes, which you've chopped, and the insides of the eggplants. Mash the garlic very finely and add it to the mixture along with the chopped parsley. Simmer for five minutes.

Now stuff the mixture into the eggplant shells, cut the remaining four tomatoes and the mozzarella cheese into slices, and divide these among the eggplant halves, putting the cheese on first and then topping it with the tomatoes. Sprinkle each eggplant with herbal seasoning, pepper, and basil, and drizzle each with a little water. Bake for forty-five minutes and serve warm or cold.

BENEFIT: Eggplant Entire contains vitamins E and K and some of the vitamin B complex, as well as the minerals calcium, manganese, phosphorus, selenium, sulfur, and some iodine. It also provides protein from the cheese.

The vitamin E, selenium, and sulfur in this dish make your skin youthful and elastic, while the iodine and calcium are wonderful for lustrous hair.

ZESTFUL ZUCCHINI

    4 *large zucchini*
$1/2$ *pound calves' liver, cut in small pieces*
    2 *onions, peeled and chopped*
    1 *egg, beaten*
    4 *tablespoons chopped parsley*
    4 *tablespoons brown rice, cooked*
    1 *tablespoon Parmesan cheese*
    2 *tablespoons whole-wheat crumbs*
    4 *tomatoes, chopped*
    3 *tablespoons olive oil*
      herbal seasoning and pepper

Preheat the oven to 350°.

Cook the zucchini in boiling salted water for two minutes. Cut them in half lengthwise; spoon out the insides. You may discard these or save them for a vegetable soup.

Sauté the liver and onions until the liver loses its pink color and the onions are transparent. Mix all the other ingredients together except the crumbs and Parmesan, add this mixture to liver and onion mixture, season them with herbal seasoning and pepper, and let them simmer for another five minutes. Then divide the mixture among the zucchini halves that you've placed in a lightly greased baking dish. Sprinkle crumbs and Parmesan cheese on top and drizzle the zucchini with olive oil. Bake for thirty minutes.

Serve Zestful Zucchini with a mixed green salad and whole-grain bread.

This dish contains vitamins A, D, E, K, and lots of vitamin B complex. In addition, it provides protein and the minerals calcium, copper, chromium, iodine, iron, manganese, phosphorus, potassium, selenium, sulfur, and zinc.

BENEFIT: Zestful Zucchini is highly concentrated beauty eating: vitamins A and E and the minerals selenium, sulfur, and zinc are great skin and hair beautifiers.

BROCCOLI BOUNTY

SERVES FOUR

1 *head broccoli, separated into flowerets*
2 *tablespoons whole-wheat bread crumbs*
1 *teaspoon olive oil*
  herbal seasoning

Toast the bread crumbs lightly in olive oil and stir in herbal seasoning. Set aside. Wash the broccoli flowerets and either cook them in your steamer or directly in a half-inch of boiling water. Cook the broccoli just until tender; it should still be a deep green color. Drain it, if you've cooked it in water, and sprinkle with the crumb mixture.

BENEFIT: Broccoli Bounty is a powerhouse of nutrients. The broccoli itself has vitamin C, vitamin A, some members of the vitamin B complex, calcium, and fiber. There are more fiber and B vitamins in the whole-wheat crumbs and vitamin E in the olive oil. It's excellent for your immune system and your skin, hair, and nails.

SQUASH BOOST

2 *medium or 3 small yellow (summer) squash*

3 *tablespoons grated Parmesan cheese*

3/4 *teaspoon thyme*

Wash squash and cut each horizontally to make four or five long slices. Lay them on a baking sheet, sprinkle with cheese and thyme, and carefully pour enough water to cover the bottom of baking sheet but not to wet the top of squash. Bake at 375° for ten minutes, until cheese is melted and bubbly.

BENEFIT: Lots of vitamin A here, and calcium as well. This side dish will help keep your skin clear and your teeth strong.

PEPPERS TRICOLORE

2 *red peppers*

2 *yellow peppers*

2 *green peppers*

2 *teaspoons olive oil*

1 *clove garlic, peeled*

1/4 *teaspoon oregano*

Wash peppers and cut in thin strips, or use large shredder blade of food processor. Heat olive oil in heavy frying pan, gently sauté garlic clove until it's golden, then remove and discard. Add peppers, stir fry quickly until they've changed color but are still crisp. Sprinkle with oregano and serve.

Peppers Tricolore can be served hot, at room temperature, or cold, as a side dish or a light first course.

BENEFIT: It's full of vitamins A and C and is wonderful for your skin.

SESAME ASPARAGUS

1 *pound asparagus*

2 *tablespoons sesame seeds, toasted in frying pan*
   herbal seasoning

Cut the ends off the asparagus and wash. Place asparagus in vegetable steamer and add a half-inch of water. Season water with herbal seasoning. Steam until crisp tender. Sprinkle with toasted sesame seeds.

BENEFIT: The asparagus and sesame seeds in this simply prepared vegetable are full of fiber and give you vitamin A and some of the vitamin B complex as well. This dish is another skin and hair beautifier.

Sweet Temptations

"No, You Needn't Feel Guilty After Every Dessert"

It's satisfying to finish a meal with something sweet and it's equally satisfying to get up from the table without feeling guilty for having succumbed to temptation. (On the other hand, when you're eating for beauty as a lifelong commitment, it would be pretty unrealistic not to indulge in your favorite baroque dessert now and then. So forget about feeling guilty.) The desserts in this section will make your sweet tooth happy and still provide you with lots of beauty components, because they're made mostly of fresh and dried fruit, whole-grain products, yoghurt, cottage cheese, and beaten egg whites.

STRAWBERRY SMOOTHIE

SERVES THREE TO FOUR

2 pints ripe strawberries, washed and hulled

3 egg whites, stiffly beaten

3 tablespoons low-fat cottage cheese

1 tablespoon raw sugar

juice of 1/2 lemon

a little artificial sweetener if the strawberries aren't sweet enough

2 tablespoons slivered almonds

Mash the strawberries with the cottage cheese, sugar, and lemon juice and then fold in the stiffly beaten egg whites. Garnish with slivered almonds and serve immediately.

BENEFIT: Strawberry Smoothie gives you vitamins A, C, D, K, and lots of the vitamin B complex, as well as the minerals calcium, magnesium, manganese, phosphorus, selenium, sulfur, and zinc. It contains almost no fat and very little sugar, and it's wonderful for smooth, velvety skin.

BANANA BOUNCE

4 *ripe bananas*
2 *egg whites, stiffly beaten*
$1/4$ *cup dates, finely chopped*
$1/4$ *cup walnuts, chopped*
2 *tablespoons low-fat cottage cheese*
$2/3$ *cup low-fat yoghurt*
artificial sweetener, to taste

Mash bananas with cottage cheese and yoghurt, fold in the dates and nuts, and add a little artificial sweetener, if necessary. Fold in the stiffly beaten egg whites and garnish with nuts.

BENEFIT: Banana Bounce contains vitamins A, D, E, K, and some of the vitamin B complex, as well as the minerals calcium, iron, magnesium, manganese, phosphorus, potassium, selenium, sulfur, and zinc.

Since calcium, magnesium, manganese, selenium, and potassium produce base compounds, while phosphorus and sulfur produce acids, Banana Bounce helps to maintain the body's acid-base balance and protects against hyperacidity. This is especially good for the skin, because hyperacidity can lead to dryness and aging. Our digestion also benefits from the fiber in the bananas, nuts, and dates and from the bacteria in the yoghurt.

FRUIT SURPRISE

2 *firm pears*

2 *firm peaches*

4 *apricots, chopped*

1/3 *cup whole–wheat crumbs*

1/4 *cup raw sugar*

1 *ounce butter*

1/4 *cup low–fat cottage cheese*

1 *ounce slivered almonds*

Cut the pears and peaches in half and remove seeds and pits. Scoop out a little of the inside and mix it with the chopped apricots, crumbs, cottage cheese, sugar, and half of the butter. Pile this mixture on the fruit halves, sprinkle with slivered almonds, dot with the remaining butter, and broil until the almonds are brown and crisp.

BENEFIT: Vitamins A, C, D, E, F, K, and some of the vitamin B complex are contained in the Fruit Surprise, as well as calcium, chromium, iron, magnesium, manganese, phosphorus, potassium, and zinc. This dessert is wonderful for youthful skin, strong and healthy nails and teeth, and gleaming hair.

PINEAPPLE TREAT

$^1/_2$ cup whole-wheat flour

1 level teaspoon baking powder

2 eggs, beaten

$^1/_4$ cup butter

1 small pineapple

$^1/_4$ cup raw sugar

$^1/_3$ cup low-fat cottage cheese

Peel the pineapple and cut it into small pieces. Preheat the oven to 350°.

Cream the butter and sugar until they are fluffy, add the beaten eggs, and then stir in the flour and the baking powder. Fold in half of the chopped pineapple and bake the mixture in a lightly greased eight-inch cake pan for twenty-five to thirty minutes, or until the surface of the cake springs back when lightly touched. Cool for about half an hour and then turn the cake out on a pretty plate.

Beat the cottage cheese until it's smooth and then fold in the remainder of the chopped pineapple. When the torte is completely cool, cut it in half horizontally. Spread the bottom half with the cottage cheese and pineapple mixture and replace the top half. Dust the top lightly with confectioner's sugar.

BENEFIT: Pineapple Treat provides the vitamins A, B, C, D, E, and K, and the minerals copper, chromium, iron, magnesium, manganese, phosphorus, potassium, selenium, sodium, sulfur, and zinc.

With all of those vitamins and minerals, Pineapple Treat is wonderful for beautifying your hair and skin and for strengthening your immune system.

BERRY PUDDING

1/2 pint strawberries

1/2 pint raspberries

1/2 pint blackberries

1/2 pint each black and red currants (these may be difficult to get, but you can either double some of the above varieties or substitute blueberries)

1/4 cup raw sugar

8–10 slices of whole wheat sponge cake

Wash all of the fruit, drain it, and then cook it in a large pot over low heat for five minutes. Drain the cooked berries (refrigerate the liquid; it's a delicious vitamin-packed drink) and mix them with the sugar. Line a two-quart mold or baking dish with part of the sponge cake, put the fruit on top of the cake, and cover it with the remaining cake slices. Weight down the cake with a heavy plate and refrigerate it overnight. The next day, turn it out of the mold and decorate the pudding with yoghurt cream (1/2 cup yoghurt beaten with 1 teaspoon sugar and a little vanilla extract).

BENEFIT: Berry Pudding contains lots of vitamin C, some vitamin B complex, and vitamins E and F. It also has calcium, copper, chromium, iron, manganese, potassium, zinc, and lots of fiber. The vitamin C makes for radiant skin, and all that fiber is great for your digestion. The yoghurt cream is a beauty bonus that contains vitamins A, D, and vitamin B complex, in addition to calcium and phosphorus.

FRUITY BEAUTY

S E R V E S   F O U R   T O   S I X

- 1 honeydew melon
- 1 orange
- 1 tangerine
- 1 apple
- 1 pear
- 1 banana
- 1/2 pound grapes
- 1 small pineapple
- juice of 1 lemon
- 1 tablespoon raw sugar

Wash and peel the fruit (except for the apple, pear, and grapes) and cut all of it into bite-sized pieces. Mix these pieces with sugar and lemon juice. Refrigerate and serve with yoghurt cream, if desired.

BENEFIT: There's lots of vitamin C and also vitamin A in Fruity Beauty. Besides that, it's very high in fiber.

Fruity Beauty is especially good for blemish free skin and good eyesight. The high vitamin A and C content gives a boost to your immune system.

APRICOT PLEASURE

1 1/2 pounds ripe apricots
1/2 cup raw sugar
1 teaspoon cinnamon
juice of 1/2 lemon

Pie dough:

1 cup whole-wheat flour
2 ounces butter
3-4 tablespoons cold water
1/4 cup low-fat cottage cheese

Preheat the oven to 375°.

Cut the apricots in half, remove the pits, and mix the fruit with the cinnamon, sugar, and lemon juice. Place this mixture in a nine-inch pie plate.

Make the dough by cutting the butter and cottage cheese into the flour and adding a few tablespoons of cold water to form a pastry. Chill this dough in the refrigerator for about thirty minutes. Then roll it out onto a floured board until it will fit the pie pan, allowing about an inch of overlap all around the edge. Place the dough over the fruit in the pie plate and prick the dough with a fork. Bake for forty minutes. Serve warm or cold with yoghurt cream.

BENEFIT: Apricot Pleasure has vitamins A, D, E, and K, and some vitamin B complex, and the minerals calcium, copper, iron, magnesium, manganese, phosphorus, potassium, and zinc. It has lots of fiber, too.

This dessert is wonderful for clear eyes and soft, smooth skin. The vitamin A in the cottage cheese and apricots prevents dryness and hypersensitivity of the skin and protects it against blemishes.

LEMON-KIWI SORBET

S E R V E S   T H R E E

   1 cup water
   1 cup raw sugar
 3/4 cup lemon juice
   2 kiwis, peeled and mashed
     grated rind of 1 lemon
   3 egg whites, stiffly beaten

Cook the water and the sugar over low heat until the sugar is entirely dissolved. Allow this liquid to cool. Then, stir the lemon juice, kiwi purée, and lemon rind into the sugar-water mixture. Pour it all into a freezer tray, and freeze the mixture for about one hour until the liquid at the edges is frozen. Take it out of the freezer, mix it thoroughly, add the beaten egg whites, and then freeze it for two or three more hours.

BENEFIT: Lemon-Kiwi Sorbet contains vitamins A, B_2, C, D, E, and K and the minerals magnesium, potassium, selenium, and zinc. It's especially good for your skin and immune system.

This is a basic recipe that you can vary to suit your favorite fruit or fruit combinations. Try it with raspberries, bananas, peaches, melons, or whatever appeals to you the most.

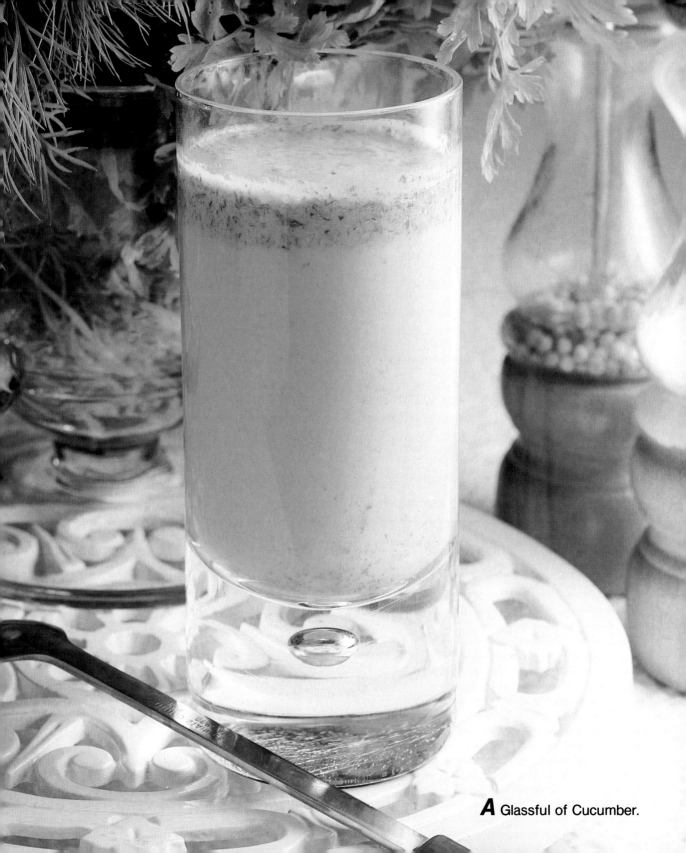

A Glassful of Cucumber.

BANANA LUSCIOUS

SERVES SIX TO EIGHT

3 large, ripe bananas, peeled and mashed

1¹/4 cups whole-wheat flour mixed with 1 level teaspoon baking powder

1 teaspoon cinnamon

¹/2 teaspoon nutmeg

³/4 cup raisins

³/4 cup dates

3 tablespoons bran

³/4 cup low-fat milk

³/4 cup chopped walnuts

Preheat the oven to 325°. Mix the mashed bananas with the flour, bran, spices, dried fruit, and nuts. Add the milk and mix thoroughly. Put the mixture into a lightly greased loaf pan and bake for one hour.

BENEFIT: Banana Luscious contains vitamins A, D, E, F, K, and nearly the entire vitamin B complex. In addition, it provides calcium, chromium, iron, magnesium, manganese, phosphorus, potassium, zinc, and lots of fiber.

All of these vitamins and minerals are good for youthful, clear skin and strong teeth. If you can't eat Beauty Meusli in the morning, then eat a piece of Banana Luscious for dessert at lunch or dinner.

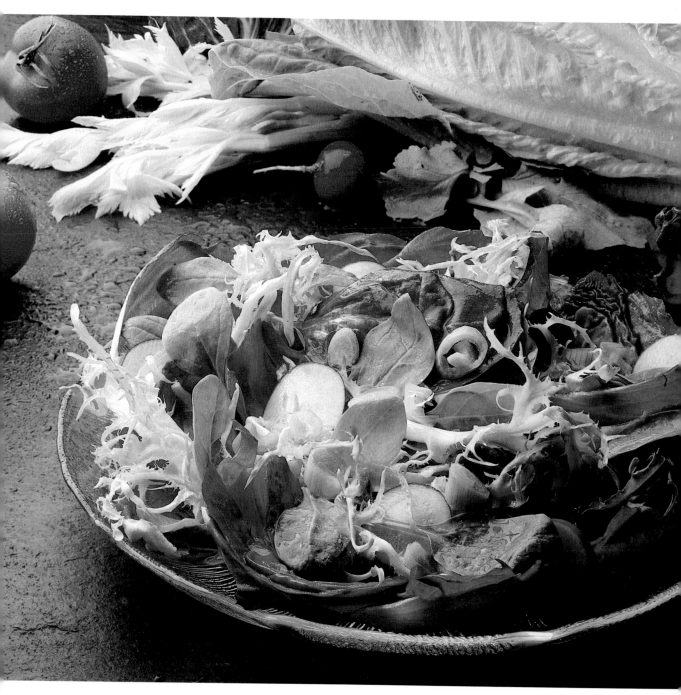

Beauty Greens (and reds),
a wonderful source of vitamin A.

RHUBARB MOUSSE

    2 *pounds rhubarb*
$1/2$ *cup sugar*
    1 *cup low-fat yoghurt*
    2 *egg whites, stiffly beaten*
      grated rind of 1 orange
    1 *level teaspoon gelatin,*
      dissolved in $1/2$ *cup hot water*

Wash rhubarb and cut it into small pieces. Combine the rhubarb with the sugar and a little water and cook it over low heat until it is soft. Allow it to cool. Mix the cooled rhubarb purée with the yoghurt, orange peel, and gelatin. Fold in the stiffly beaten egg whites. Refrigerate for about six hours to allow the mousse to set.

BENEFIT: Rhubarb Mousse contains vitamins A, B_2, D, E, and K, as well as calcium, phosphorus, selenium, sulfur, and lots of fiber.

This is a refreshing, creamy dessert that benefits your hair and skin.

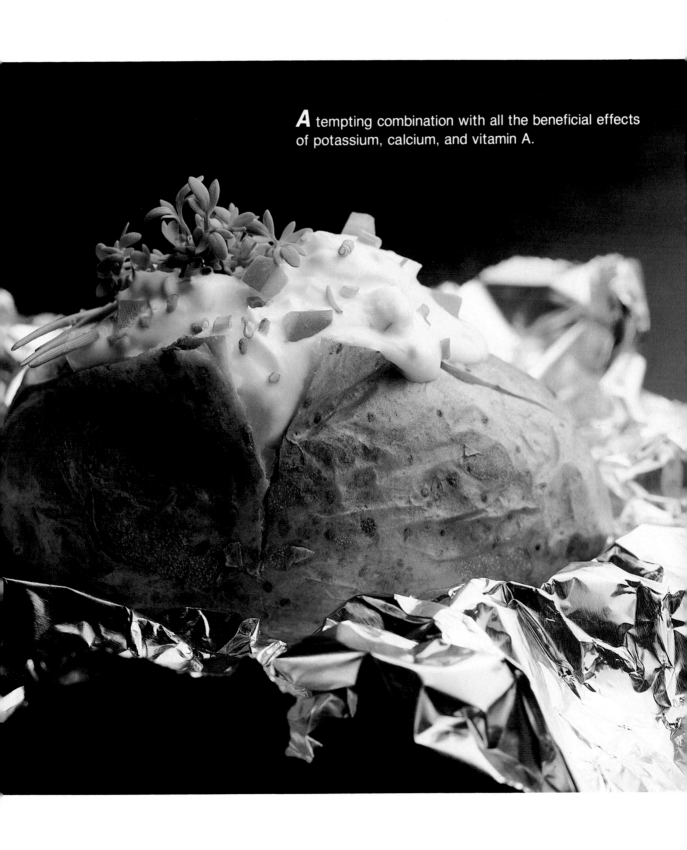

A tempting combination with all the beneficial effects of potassium, calcium, and vitamin A.

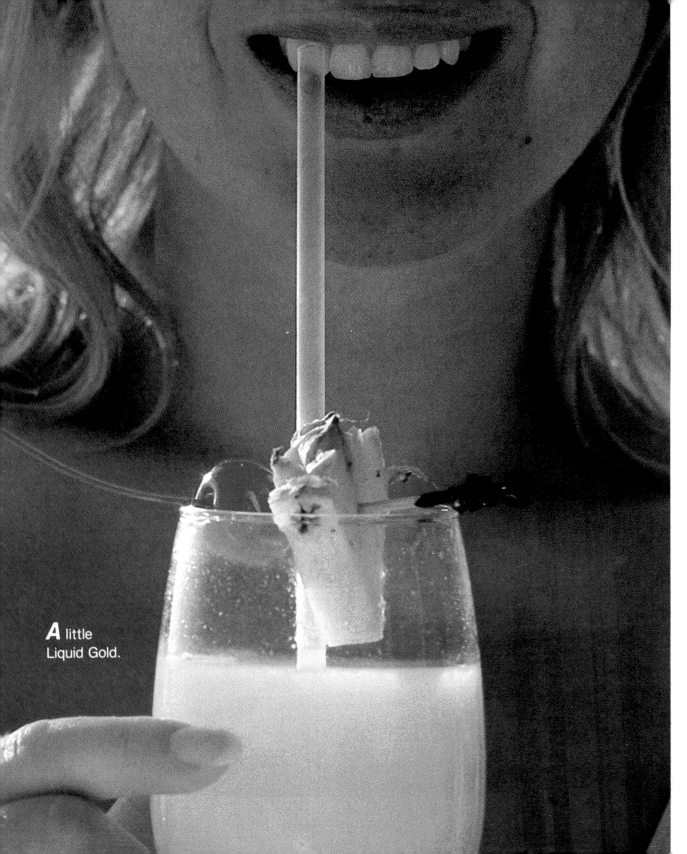

A little
Liquid Gold.

ALMOND KISSES

1 1/2 *cups ground almonds*
1/2 *cup sesame seeds*
4 *egg whites, stiffly beaten*
1/4 *cup raw sugar*
a little skim milk to make the mixture stick together
20 *whole almonds for decoration*

Preheat the oven to 375°. Mix the ground almonds, sesame seeds, sugar, and a little milk to make a paste. Carefully fold in the beaten egg whites. Grease a sheet of waxed paper lightly and put it on a baking sheet. Drop tablespoons of the mixture on the lined baking sheet so that there are twenty Almond Kisses, top each with a whole almond, and bake them for fifteen to twenty minutes, being careful not to let the bottoms get brown.

BENEFIT: Almond Kisses contain vitamins A, D, E, F, K, and almost all of the vitamin B complex. In addition, the kisses provide calcium, magnesium, manganese, potassium, sulfur, and zinc. The unsaturated fatty acids (vitamin F) in the almonds are especially good for glowing skin and lustrous hair.

Now, after telling you about all of this wonderful food that is so great for you, we're going to tell you about a few things that detract from eating for beauty. You'll find them in the next chapter, Beauty Spoilers.

The Beauty Spoilers

Choosing the right foods and serving them attractively will help you look your most beautiful. But adopting good habits is not enough. You also have to overcome bad habits. That's not easy in our overcivilized way of life today. We're faced with temptations everywhere we turn, and these temptations are generally bad for health and beauty potential. The very social fabric of our business and personal schedules encourages indulgence in the no-nos that we must avoid.

By keeping your mind firmly set on your goal of achieving a more beautiful you, you can summon up the willpower to politely refuse those foods and habits that are bad for you. In the next chapter, we'll outline some very specific strategies for choosing what is beneficial and rejecting what is destructive. This chapter discusses the dangerous foods and tells you what to avoid and why. Once you know why you must avoid certain foods and habits, saying no will be much easier.

Alcohol

Not all of the beauty no-nos are foods that you must completely avoid. Alcohol is an example of where moderation can substitute for abstinence. Alcohol shouldn't be used as a thirst-quencher. But if you sip it slowly, savoring each sip, a glass of wine to prolong relaxation after work or a pint of beer to refresh after an afternoon of skiing can be an acceptable pleasure. They will add calories that you have to subtract somewhere else in your meal planning, but neither your health nor appearance will be harmed. Be sure, however, to eat a well-balanced meal soon after you have a drink. According to Dr. Boris Tabakoff of the University of Illinois Medical Center in Chicago "alcohol depletes the system of vitamins very fast."

That glass or two of wine or mug of beer should be the outside limit. If you drink too much, your body will tell you that you're not being careful and your looks will tell everyone else.

Like caffeine and nicotine, alcohol becomes addictive when consumed in large quantities. Drinking too much greatly reduces the efficiency of the circulatory system, which can result in brain cells dying from oxygen starvation.

Moreover, alcohol attacks and irreparably damages the liver, the only organ with the capacity to break down and detoxify alcohol. The liver performs this task properly when presented with small amounts of alcohol, but when excessive drinking occurs, the organ can't function properly. Active liver cells become totally useless; they degenerate into fatty tissue, robbing the liver of a significant portion of its capacity to act as the body's own "detox" unit.

Of course, alcohol is not the only toxic material assaulting our bodies. A liver partially destroyed by too much alcohol can no longer deal with these other toxins as it should. These other materials then clog up the body, interfering with metabolism and causing problems ranging from bad breath to pasty-looking skin.

Drinking too much alcohol also steals vitamins B and C from the body, both of which are necessary for general well-being, immunity against disease, and a glowing, young-looking skin.

Cigarettes

Unlike drinking, cigarette smoking is NOT something that can be done in moderation, simply because virtually no one can. Smokers simply do not have a couple of cigarettes at special moments during the week. They either smoke a lot or quit entirely. And since smoking a lot is very destructive to your health and beauty, the only solution is to consider cigarettes an absolute no-no.

The health dangers of smoking are so well known—and so well publicized in public service ads and in complaints from non-smoking colleagues—that there's no need to recite them here. The extremely high correlation between smoking and deaths from lung cancer is, after all, no coincidence.

But the consequences of smoking on your looks are less well known. Perhaps if they are understood completely, vanity can accomplish what health concerns do not. If so, that's all to the good.

Skin is the component most vulnerable to damage from smoking, because cigarettes steal vitamin C, which is absolutely essential for maintaining healthy collagen and smooth, young-looking skin.

In addition, the carbon monoxide present in cigarette smoke attacks the walls of our blood vessels. Looking at them under a microscope, you can actually see how the smooth surface of a healthy blood vessel is roughened by carbon monoxide, creating areas susceptible to arterial deposits. In addition, carbon monoxide combines with hemoglobin, the blood's oxygen carrier, greatly reducing the blood's capacity for carrying oxygen to the organs.

Again, you see this oxygen starvation in your skin, which will wrinkle prematurely and look dry and lifeless. Remember that the same kind of deterioration from reduced oxygen is happening to your internal organs.

Caffeine

You ought to avoid coffee and tea just as completely as you avoid cigarettes. The caffeine in coffee and tea (where the chemical analog is technically known as theine) is addictive, just as nicotine is. While there's no doubt that a glass of wine or beer can be an important component of the unwinding so essential for a busy person's healthy life, there are so many completely acceptable alternatives to caffeine-laden drinks that there's no reason to take even the modest health risks involved.

Rather than "real" tea, sip an herbal brew. There are a large variety on the market, and you can find a blend of peppermint, rosehip, chamomile, black currant, hibiscus, apple, or cinnamon that will fit your personal taste. And rather than coffee, choose one of the grain substitutes made from barley or rye, a chicory blend, or, if you must, a chemically decaffeinated coffee. Now that all the major cola makers offer a caffeine-free diet alternative to their basic formulation, there's no good reason for choosing the caffeinated Cokes or Pepsis.

Any of these substitutes will avoid the concentrated stimulants that speed up your heartbeat, increase the acidity in your stomach, and make your nerves feel taut.

You know that when you drink too much coffee, tea, or cola, you are overstimulated; you overreact; and you are apt to be too startled at noises, bright lights, and minor irritations you later wish you had handled without losing your cool. That same overreaction keeps your mind flitting from subject to subject at night, keeping you awake and robbing your body of rejuvenating sleep. Longer term, you can expect stomach ulcers and a disruption in metabolic function from continued overindulgence.

So vow now to cut out the caffeine.

Salt

There's simply too much salt in the normal American diet. Would you believe that our national consumption works out to fifteen pounds a year for every man, woman, and child in this country!

The sodium content of normal table salt is dangerous; too much can lead directly to high blood pressure, and can cause a heart attack or a stroke. "Hypertension is very much a disease of the Western world. It is almost unheard of in 'primitive' societies where salt is not a common food additive," notes Dr. Sheldon Saul Hendler, a biochemist and physician who teaches at the University of California's San Diego campus.

The link between salt consumption and high blood pressure is not a worry for everyone. Some are at risk and some are not. But since medical science has yet to find a way to warn us whether we are in the high-risk group, it is best to avoid salt.

You cannot, of course, control the amount of salt added to processed foods or to what you eat away from your own home. So try to counteract the sodium intake by eating plenty of calcium-rich foods such as skimmed milk products, fish, and leafy green vegetables. By lowering your blood pressure, the calcium helps counteract the deleterious effects of the sodium.

Too much salt in our diet leads to water retention, causing joints, legs, and hands to swell and eyes to look puffy. Use a low-sodium salt or an herbal blend salt substitute in your cooking. See how long you can make a shaker last. It's better to wean yourself from salt entirely, and learn to appreciate the true taste of the foods you eat.

Fats

Just as our bodies need sugar, they need fats. But a normal diet provides the amount we need—a very small quantity—without any fat-heavy foods (like red meat) and anything deep-fried, which we are better off avoiding. Fish, nuts, cereals, and dairy products give us all the fat we need.

Eating excessive fats is the quickest route to obesity and to straining the biological system that was designed for a normal weight body. What's excessive? Consuming more than one-quarter of your daily caloric intake in the form of fats.

Obesity is only the beginning of the beauty and health toll taken by ingesting too much fat. It can lead to cancer, especially colorectal cancer. A 1983 article in the *International Journal of Cancer* reported the results of a comparison of one hundred people in Athens, Greece, who ate meat-heavy, high fat diets with an equal number of people from the same city who ate little meat and lots of vegetables. The result: Those who favored meat were eight times as likely to develop colorectal cancer as those who seldom ate it.

No one yet knows for sure why a high-fat diet seems to encourage development of cancer. But *New York Times* science writer Jane Brody outlines what is currently deemed the most likely explanation: "During the metabolism of fats and cholesterol, substances are formed that are cancer-promoting, including some chemicals that mimic the action of sex hormones, which are notorious for their ability to stimulate the growth of cancers."

In addition, fat can cause heart disease. It can aggravate a predisposition to high blood pressure, diabetes, arthritis, gout, arteriosclerosis.

Too much fat in your diet will show on your skin; it will be greasy, unattractive from a distance, and not very pretty up close.

Sugar

Be it white, golden brown, or dark brown, sugar in anything but minute quantities is bad news for good looks. Our bodies can make good use of sugar when, as a naturally-occuring component of fruit or milk products, it is digested slowly and made available to the pancreas in very small quantities. But when we eat cookies or buttercreams, the pancreas is overloaded and reacts by producing large quantities of insulin to process the sugar.

If this happens many times a day, the pancreas learns to expect such onslaughts. Constant overindulgence in sugar-rich foods will cause the pancreas to produce increased quantities of insulin whenever you eat something sweet. At worst, you can develop diabetes. Even if you don't, you may find yourself short-tempered and often fatigued beyond what you would expect. You know that eating sweets even in moderation will make you gain weight, often in the places where it will be least flattering. You are also likely to develop blotchy skin, because overdoing your sugar intake upsets the careful balance of nutrients vital to beauty and causes deficiencies, particularly of the vitamin B complex.

Occasional desserts are alright; your body can deal with the piece of birthday cake or the Belgian chocolate that your boss brought back for his staff. But then go back to your beauty-making routine. If it's abandoned for too long, it really will show.

Those, then, are the six no-nos. Each is bad for you, but in combination they can be even worse. For instance, Dr. M. Ward Hinds conducted research at the Cancer Center of Hawaii that showed that smokers with diets high in fats have a lung cancer rate that is even higher than that for smokers who watch their fat intake. And research results published in the *American Journal of Clinical Nutrition* show that the chances of salt bringing on hypertension are significantly higher in persons who also consume large quantities of sugar.

So curb your alcohol intake. Stop smoking. Opt for caffeine-free drinks. Stay away from refined sugar. Select a diet with only small amounts of salt and fat. And then stand in front of your mirror and take pleasure in how terrific you look!

CHAPTER FOUR

Strategies for Lifelong Beauty

To stay beautiful, you've got to incorporate the beauty foods into your daily life; the occasional carrot stick won't do it. That won't be difficult to do once you've seen the results.

The most important foods are those in your refrigerator and those you reach for first when you're hungry and want a snack.

Lifelong beauty strategies are not nearly as restrictive as you might imagine. They just take a little organization and desire to be beautiful.

The next time you go grocery shopping, take a good look at your shopping cart and keep the following points in mind.

- Replace white-flour foods and white rice with whole-grain products and brown rice. Almost nothing in white flour makes you beautiful because all of the fiber and nearly all of the essential beauty vitamins have been lost in the refining process. Your basic carbohydrates are whole-grain breads and crackers, although you can have a little white-flour bread occasionally.

- Leave light and heavy cream, half-and-half, and fatty cheeses in the dairy case and buy low-fat or skim milk (whole milk in tea and coffee substitutes is okay if that's all that's available), low-fat cottage cheese and yoghurt, and farmer cheeses, such as mozzarella, are good too.

- Instead of chocolate, cookies, cakes, and candy, go on a fruit shopping binge. You can also lay in a supply of fresh and dried fruit, unsalted nuts, and whole-grain cookies.

- Eggs, fish, poultry, and lean meat should definitely be in your cart.

- Vegetables are it! They're one of your chief beauty sources because they're full of vitamins and low in calories. Have a good selection of fresh vegetables and crisp salad ingredients in your refrigerator.

- You can buy small quantities of butter; but whenever you can, try to substitute other similar products with less cholesterol and fewer calories. In cooking, use vegetable oils and try fat-free methods.

- Replace jams and preserves that are more than half sugar with the sugar-free variety. Or you might want to try making your own from fresh or dried fruits.

- Stock up on mineral water and natural fruit juices so that you can feel beautiful while you're quenching your thirst.

If your kitchen is well supplied with beauty foods and you've given your last candy bar to the neighbors, you're well on your way. Then you'll automatically reach for yoghurt with fresh fruit in your refrigerator. For other snacks, try crisp raw vegetables with a cottage cheese dip and some whole-grain crackers. When you want more than a snack, try a hearty slice of whole-grain toast with cottage cheese, tomatoes, and herbal seasoning. Have dried fruit and whole-grain cookies instead of a rich dessert and then you can get up from the table feeling virtuous. Your little repast was not only delicious, but good for you as well. No worries about blemishes, dull hair, or gaining weight. Quite the contrary. The more often you pass up the marbled roast beef, fries, and chocolate cake for such beauty foods as fish, fruit salads, and whole-grain breads, the better the effect. You'll look radiant and feel great.

Beauty at Home

While devising my lifelong beauty strategies, I discovered ways to get around some of my bad habits with little tricks to ensure a variety of good-tasting foods that aren't expensive. I'd like to pass them on to you.

YOU DON'T HAVE TO GIVE UP SWEETS. As you know from the section on Sweet Temptations, you can *Eat Yourself Beautiful* and still enjoy sweets.

On a day-to-day basis, you should replace sugar, which is a high-calorie, low-vitamin no-no with other sweet goodies that aren't bad for you.*

Honey is one of the best alternatives. It's very sweet, which means you can use less, it contains small amounts of many beauty vitamins and minerals, and it consists entirely of fructose, which has fewer calories than sucrose—conventional sugar. Fructose also is easier for our bodies to process because it does not involve the pancreas as much as refined sugar. Because it has a higher concentration of "sweetness," you need less. Although it's better for you, honey still contains almost as many calories as sugar, therefore it should be used in moderation. Another excellent alternative to sugar is fresh or dried fruit. Fruit contains many beauty vitamins and minerals as well as fiber. Depending on the season, you can have apricots, peaches, grapes, pears, or, for more exotic tastes, mangoes and papayas for dessert.

Dried fruit is especially good for a sweet tooth because it's sweeter than fresh. It's always available and doesn't spoil as quickly as fresh fruit, making it an excellent alternative to sugary desserts.

*Some of the recipes in this book call for raw sugar because of its bulk. The recipe will not work without it and the amount is small. But, in general, you should always try to substitute harmless, low-calorie artificial sweeteners in your diet, whenever possible.

Dried apricots, pears, dates, or figs are delicious. Just pour boiling water over the fruit and let it stand overnight. The next day, purée it and store it in glass jars. To make it even sweeter, use a little artificial sweetener, which in *small* quantities is not bad for you.

If you do without refined sugar for a couple of weeks and have only fruit, fruit juices, and honey, you won't even want that excessively sugary taste, one of the keys to eating yourself beautiful.

YOU DON'T HAVE TO EAT BLAND FOOD. We
said in previous chapters that table salt is bad for your health and your beauty. The sodium in table salt causes elevated blood pressure making you more susceptible to strokes and heart attacks. High salt consumption also causes water retention, which results in unsightly swelling of the joints, legs, and hands.

There are many alternative seasonings that can make avoiding salt easier. Low-sodium diet salt is one logical alternative (but make sure you check with your doctor before using it). You might also consider pepper, mustard, paprika, soy sauce (not too much because it is salty), and all sorts of tasty herbs and spices. Vegetable bouillon cubes or vegetable concentrate can be used for soups, stews, and cooked meat and fish dishes, as well as for vegetables, rice, and whole-grain products.

Like a desire for very sweet foods, that for very salty foods is just a habit and one you won't miss after a few weeks of low-salt eating.

INSTEAD OF FATS. Too much fat in our diet is one of the
most unhealthy eating practices in our society. Increasingly, physicians and researchers in nutrition are realizing that in addition to causing overweight and skin blemishes, excessive fat consumption and too little exercise may help to account for the high incidence of cancer, strokes, and heart attacks.

Since most of the cooking methods that use a lot of fat can easily be replaced by low-fat alternatives, you can check out the tips below for some ideas and do some experimenting in your own kitchen.

If possible, meat should not be breaded and fried, sautéed in oil, or served with heavy cream sauces. If you need a little fat, use vegetable oils and avoid fats that are solid at room temperature.

Refrigerate soups and stews before serving. That way you can skim the fat that rises to the top before you reheat the dish. Doing that turns a potential no-no into a real beauty food.

Meat can be broiled or it can be braised or simmered in vegetable stock. Fairly large pieces of meat can be roasted in the oven and allowed to make their own gravy. All visible fat should be trimmed before serving.

Fish is very well suited for fat-free preparation. It can be poached, broiled with lemon juice and pepper, or stuffed and then baked in aluminum foil. Or you can turn it into a fish stew, soup, or casserole. You can also combine cooked fish with a salad dressing and a tossed green salad and have a delicious, beauty-enhancing cold meal.

Lobster, shrimp, and mussels can be cooked in a seasoned broth and then served hot or cold with a refreshing herbed yoghurt sauce. Brown rice, whole-grain toast, and salad round out this light, easy-to-prepare meal.

The best fat-free way to prepare eggs is to boil or poach them. But you can also prepare delicious soufflés and omelettes with little or no fat. Steamed vegetables are an excellent additional ingredient for these.

Eggs contain a number of important beauty vitamins and minerals, especially vitamins A, B_2, D, and E and the minerals sulfur, zinc, iron, and phosphorus, as well as lecithin, which is part of every cell in our body. As far as its beauty contribution is concerned, lecithin helps distribute your body weight and contributes to clear, youthful skin. Also, like the vitamin B complex, lecithin is important for maintaining a healthy nervous system. Eggs also contain some unsaturated fatty acids. We've already mentioned the cholesterol content of eggs elsewhere so keep that in mind.

Vegetable dishes of all kinds are ideally suited for low-fat cooking. They can be varied in many different and delicious ways. Vegetables can be steamed, braised, topped with low-fat cheese and baked in the oven; made into curries, purées, stews, and soups; combined with rice, potatoes, fish, meat, eggs, and natural grain products such as wheat, oats, barley—like this sentence, the list is endless. Almost all of our vegetables are stocked year-round so their vitamins and fiber are always available. From bean ragout to yam soufflé, your delicious vegetable inventions will convert your family and friends into enthusiastic beauty food fans.

Salads and crudités are of course the *ne plus ultra* of your lifelong beauty strategy. They contain the most vitamins, minerals, and fiber and the fewest calories. They do the most for our beauty, health, and well-being.

Try and eat a fresh, crisp salad at least once or twice a day (more often is even better). Keep a dish of rabbit food (cucumbers, carrot sticks, radishes, cauliflower, zucchini, celery, and whatever else appeals to you) ready in your refrigerator at all times to combat the nibblies. Try your cucumber, carrot, and zucchini sticks dipped in seasoned cottage cheese.

DRINKING RIGHT IS PART OF IT TOO. Drinking a lot of liquids is essential for beauty, but they need to be the right ones.

You ought to keep away from no-nos such as coffee; strong tea; sweet, non-alcoholic beverages; and alcohol. They either raise your blood pressure or overload the pancreas with too much sugar, which causes excess insulin secretion and, in the long run, increases the probability of diabetes. Drinking sugared or alcoholic drinks regularly is definitely not part of a lifelong beauty strategy.

But you can be generous with mineral water, some of the herbal teas (check these out with your doctor because not all herbal teas are innocuous), and coffee substitutes that contain no caffeine. You should also try freshly-pressed vegetable and fruit juices and, to warm up, a vegetable bouillon cube dissolved in hot water.

Try an herb tea with lemon and honey for breakfast and a coffee substitute with milk for a pre-noontime treat. Have cold mineral water with lemon for lunch and for that all-important afternoon pick-me-up, a beauty drink of mineral water and fruit juice or buttermilk. If you're at home you can put your blender and your imagination to work to come up with a tasty treat.

Make some changes at the cocktail hour. Instead of an alcoholic drink, try some beauty in a glass—freshly squeezed vegetable or fruit juice or a cooler made of mineral water and fruit juice with a little lemon. You'll cut out loads of calories and spare your system the stress caused by alcohol that was discussed in the previous chapter. Alcohol gives you a brief feeling of being calm and relaxed, but that's followed immediately by greater fatigue and a decline in alertness.

If you're used to having a couple of glasses of wine every evening, you'll be amazed at how alert, awake, and energetic you'll feel if you drink something non-alcoholic instead. The whole trick is to have alcohol very infrequently and in small quantities. That way your body can easily deal with its negative effects and your appearance won't suffer.

The diminished oxygen supply that results from regular alcohol intake is due to constriction of blood vessels and a slight increase in density of the blood. In addition, the liver is the only organ in the body that can neutralize and decompose alcohol. If you drink a lot, it becomes overloaded and your liver cells degenerate into non-functional fatty tissue.

The outer signs of regular alcohol intake are pasty skin; a slightly red and swollen nose; and watery, cloudy eyes. But changing your drinking habits has the potential to get rid of these signs. When your liver has recovered, and depending on your earlier drinking habits it may take a few months or a few years, your skin and eyes will be clear and bright again.

BELIEVE IT OR NOT, EATING BEAUTIFULLY MAKES YOU BEAUTIFUL TOO. It may surprise you, but how you eat—whether you consciously enjoy your food or simply gulp it down—and how much you eat can have both positive and negative effects on your looks.

First, don't eat while you're doing something else, like watching TV or reading. Standing in the kitchen and nibbling isn't good either because you're not aware of enjoying your food and you can't keep track of how much you've eaten.

Every time you eat, even if it's only a snack, arrange the food attractively on a pretty plate, and don't fill the plate too full. Take very small bites and chew each one thoroughly; have an occasional sip of water.

There are a number of good reasons for these habits. We don't eat just because we're hungry. Most of us eat with our eyes, to satisfy an emotional need. Eating slowly and being aware of what we eat is the fastest way to satisfy our appetite.

Medical research has shown that chewing thoroughly starts off the digestive process in the mouth, and that our stomachs can digest food best and make optimum use of nutrients when we eat slowly. Furthermore, we don't feel really satisfied until twenty to thirty minutes after eating. This means that if you don't stop eating until you're full, you'll feel uncomfortably stuffed half an hour later. If you eat slowly you're giving yourself more of a chance to feel full with less food.

This brings us to a very important beauty tip: Try to get up from the table still feeling a little hungry. Twenty minutes later you'll be fully satisfied but you won't have overloaded your stomach with unnecessary quantities.

SHOULD IT BE WARM OR COLD? Myths about eating warm and cold food have existed for generations. For example, Austrian grandmothers would tell you that cold coffee (which is a no-no anyway) makes you beautiful; other grandmothers would say that you should have at least one hot meal daily, because it's more nourishing for your system. These myths are just that—myths.

Coffee will never make you beautiful whether it's hot or cold. What you eat is more important than the temperature of the food when you put it in your mouth. It makes a difference whether you eat vegetables raw (with all of the vitamins and fiber intact) or cooked. Whether the cooked vegetables are warm or cold has no bearing on their nutritional value since all food is at the same temperature in the stomach five minutes after you eat it. The only thing that's important is what you eat and what tastes good to you. If you're hot, drink something cold. If you need something hot to wake you up, have some hot tea every morning. The choice of hot or cold is up to you.

WHEN YOU OVERINDULGE. Few of us are absolute health freaks and we're all going to eat and drink too much occasionally when we're out with friends or home alone.

If you've been following the *Eat Yourself Beautiful* approach and practicing lifelong beauty strategies, the occasional indulgence (provided it is only occasional) doesn't matter at all. Your appearance won't suffer. A day of salads and beauty drinks is all your body needs to forget the chocolates, the mayonnaise on your fish, and all those glasses of champagne.

Gorging regularly on cakes and candy, fatty cheeses, and alcohol will make your skin look dull and will make you feel bloated. Obviously, overindulgence won't allow you to look your best.

But when you are going to overindulge, do it consciously and enjoy every last bite and sip. Don't spoil the enjoyment with a guilty conscience. You've done it and now you'll go back to beauty eating. Neither your body nor your face will suffer! No guilt trips, please, because feeling good about yourself is one of *the* most important beauty precepts.

Beauty When You're Out

Your beauty strategies are not limited to when you're home. Here are a few tricks for when you're at the office, traveling, or eating in restaurants or when you've been invited out for meals.

AT THE OFFICE. If you can't go to a restaurant or cafeteria for lunch and you're limited to a sandwich, don't worry. It takes only a few minutes before you leave the house to pack a salad with dressing on the side and a whole-grain roll, a container of cottage cheese with soybean sprouts and sesame seeds, or one of the following beauty sandwiches. You might also like some fresh fruit and some of the raw vegetables that you keep in the refrigerator for snacks.

BEAUTY SANDWICHES. Make each sandwich with two slices of whole-grain bread spread with a thin layer of farmer's cheese to which you've added herbal seasoning.

CHICKEN

1 small tomato, thinly sliced
6 slices of cucumber
4 lettuce leaves
1 teaspoon mild mustard
2 ounces cooked chicken, skin removed

ASPARAGUS

2 asparagus spears, cooked, seasoned with herbal
seasoning and pepper, and cut in pieces
8 slices of cucumber
1 tablespoon yoghurt dressing
about 10 cooked shrimp

VEGETABLE

2 flowerets broccoli, cooked and cut
2 lettuce leaves
1 walnut, chopped coarsely
1 heaping teaspoon cottage cheese

EGG

1 hard-boiled egg, cut in slices
8 slices of cucumber
4 tomato slices
herbal seasoning, pepper, and paprika

SMOKED SALMON

(as a special treat)

2 thin slices smoked salmon
juice of $1/4$ lemon
6 slices of cucumber
pepper

RESTAURANT EATING. It's easy to *Eat Yourself Beautiful* in restaurants. Most of them don't mind making minor changes, such as broiling foods instead of sautéing and serving salad without heavy, creamy dressings. All you have to do is keep in mind the beauty foods that you can eat until ordering them becomes second nature for you. Your first course can be any clear soup such as consommé, oxtail, or turtle soup. You can have vegetable soups as long as they're prepared without cream (or with a little bit of light cream). Cold first courses can be any kind of salad, which is full of vitamins, or shrimp or other seafood (without heavy cocktail sauces; use lemon juice and black pepper, or a little vinaigrette or yoghurt dressing). Because of its relatively high fat content, smoked salmon is advisable only in small quantities.

Mozzarella with tomatoes, artichoke hearts with vinaigrette sauce, melon, or a fresh fruit salad are all wonderful starters.

For the main course, the rule is the simpler the better. You can have any kind of broiled or braised fish, meat, or poultry, accompanied by cooked vegetables without butter, salad, and rice or a baked potato. Trim all visible fat and stay away from vegetables in cream sauce, fried rice, scalloped potatoes, tartar sauce on fish, and herbed butter sauces. Instead, stick with beauty foods, such as lean meat or broiled shrimp, fish, and chicken accompanied by vegetable salads and rice.

Don't eat dessert just out of habit. And don't feel that you have to order food you don't want to eat to keep your friends company while they splurge. But if your appetite and associates do demand it, there are desserts you can have that won't jeopardize your looks or your vitamin intake.

First of all there's fruit; any fresh fruit such as strawberries, raspberries, pineapple, or kiwis are wonderful. They have lots of vitamins and fiber, very little sugar, and no fat. Fresh fruit salad is another good thing provided you don't eat too much of the sugar syrup. Fruit sorbet, yoghurt, and cottage cheese with fruit are also fine in small quantities. Unfortunately, there's no way to extend the beauty food label to cream, fatty cheese, chocolate mousse, or rich cakes.

If you can't escape, eat the no-nos in very small helpings so that you don't ambush your body with a lot of concentrated fat and sugar.

In general, there are a few basics for beauty-conscious eating in restaurants: Eat only as much as you want. Restaurant portions are usually too large so you can leave at least a third of the food on your plate.

Don't be forced to order or eat something you don't want for the sake of being polite. It's your body and you have to decide what you eat. It's important that you eat with enjoyment and without a guilty conscience. Everyone will understand (and perhaps be envious of or amazed at) your refusing the salad that's loaded with mayonnaise or the gooey chocolate cake. They won't think you're being impolite.

Take occasional small sips of wine to enhance the taste of your food but if you're thirsty drink tap or mineral water. A before-dinner drink can be fruit or vegetable juice instead of a cocktail. You should have after-dinner coffee only occasionally because coffee elevates your blood pressure and acts as a stimulant for your entire system. It's also very habit-forming.

Our last bit of advice is very simple. Don't salt your food. Salt increases blood pressure in most people, therefore greatly increasing the risk of strokes and—because of hypersalemia in the stomach—gastric ulcers. As we've said before, high salt intake also results in water retention which shows up as swollen arms, legs, ankles, or hands.

Cutting down on salt doesn't mean that you have to give up seasoned food. Quite the contrary. If you want to replace the salty taste (which in good cooking shouldn't be the main source of taste anyway), you can experiment with all sorts of herbs and condiments. Such experiments will lead you to expand your taste spectrum without threatening your health or your looks. After a few weeks, you won't even miss the salt.

The good news is that you can *Eat Yourself Beautiful* and still enjoy a restaurant meal that includes first, main, and dessert courses and a little wine. There are many foods to choose from. Because of the low fat and sugar content of beauty foods, you can eat a really satisfying meal and not have that overfull feeling that comes from a heavy, fatty dinner with lots of wine. You'll get up from the table feeling pleasantly full but not overloaded. Moreover, because of the even flow of energy from unrefined nutrients, such as whole-grains and vegetables, the feeling will last for many hours.

Once you've switched from fatty foods and lots of alcohol to a beauty menu, you'll be so delighted with the results—your improved appearance and the sensation of well-being—that you won't feel like going back to your former habits.

WHEN YOU'RE INVITED OUT. What happens to your beauty food approach when you're invited to someone's home and you feel politeness demands that you do justice to all the food for fear of insulting the cook? If you want to eat in a beauty-conscious way and don't want to eat all the no-nos, you'll simply have to politely decline whatever doesn't fit into your beauty diet. You could pass yourself off as a health food nut. That way, the guests

will laugh and the hostess won't feel personally responsible for your not eating.

You'll feel much better if you're the only one who doesn't eat two helpings of chocolate mousse than if you end up suffering from an overly full stomach and a guilty conscience. Regardless of where you spend the evening, be it at a cocktail party, a buffet, or a sit-down dinner, you'll probably find enough food that you can eat safely. You can eat all of the salads except those loaded with mayonnaise. All types of fish, meat, and poultry are fine, so long as you trim all visible fat from the meat and remove the skin from the poultry. You can eat a lot of poached or steamed fish as long as you don't eat any accompanying mayonnaise. Vegetables without butter are excellent as are rice and cooked potatoes. Turn down fried or scalloped potatoes because of their high fat content.

Avoid foods with heavy cream sauces and all fried foods, since both contain large quantities of fat. Politely declining them will save you from lots of beauty no-nos.

Be very careful with desserts and try to stick to fruit if you can. If it's a birthday party or some other celebration, take a piece of cake and push it around on your plate; no one will notice.

You can even handle an opulent five-course meal following these tips. Drink mineral water or juice, take small bites, and chew thoroughly. Take frequent sips of water and talk. You can get through the entire meal that way and feel pleasantly satisfied without being stuffed.

We have a few other ideas for a cocktail party or buffet.

Cocktail parties usually follow the same sequence of alcohol, peanuts, canapés, a little more alcohol (actually your glass is always full so you don't really know how much you've had), another handful of peanuts and so on. After the first half-hour, you've lost track of how many little sandwiches, peanuts, and cheese hors d'oeuvres you've nibbled and, after all that wine you've had, you probably don't care.

The myth that you can spend an evening with friends only if you eat and drink too much is just that—a myth. Any beauty and health conscious individual will tell you that's not necessary. But standing around and eating without thinking about it often results in unintended lapses.

Try and quench your thirst with mineral water or juice and decline offers of alcoholic drinks. But don't feel that you have to refuse a glass of wine for a toast.

Although peanuts contain beauty vitamins B, E, and F, and the minerals calcium, magnesium, manganese, and zinc, as well as lots of protein, those served at parties are roasted in oil or butter and are very salty. Their good nutritional components are canceled out by the no-nos fat and salt; besides that they already have lots of calories without them (five hundred thirty in four ounces of peanuts). The additional calories, all in the form of fat, then make them out of sight. So politely decline the peanuts and wine and stick with the crudités, which will keep your stomach unencumbered for the next course.

The most important trick with buffets, whether they're served formally or self-service, is to take only what you really want. Don't get carried away and take something from every passing tray.

All of these tips are aimed at allowing you to go out as much as you like without jeopardizing your beauty or your conscience. By following these suggestions, you can go out every night (don't stay out too late though), enjoy yourself, and still like what you see in your mirror next morning. Your friends will wonder how you can be so radiant when you're leading such a hectic life.

In the following chapter, we'll share a few ideas that will enhance the effects of the beauty foods you eat.

More Ways to a More Beautiful You

You can't be your best if you don't eat your best, but a proper diet alone won't do it. You have to have proper muscle tone, your eyes have to give off the sparkle that can only come from a body that is properly cared for, and to exude the self-confidence that makes others have confidence in you, you have to get the better of stress before it gets the better of you.

Now that we have talked about how to *Eat Yourself Beautiful,* we're going to focus in this chapter on three other health musts. They are the steppingstones to vitality, the heart of true beauty.

Be Active

Your body was made to be used; the biggest enemy of your muscles and tissues is inactivity. Sit around too much, ride when you can walk, choose a quiet cocktail in the corner instead of a vigorous turn out on the dance floor, and your body deteriorates. Your metabolic system slows down. You don't rid yourself of the toxins that collect in your tissues and blood vessels, impairing the blood flow and diminishing the body's oxygen supply. Your cells no longer regenerate efficiently, resulting in premature aging of your entire system.

This is such an unnecessary fate, because activity can keep you young. This doesn't mean you have to pump iron or train for a marathon. But it does mean that you have to change your habits.

From now on, one of your top priorities will be to keep your body in motion. Not hectic frenzy, just movement. Leave a little earlier for an appointment and walk instead of taking a cab. And, when you walk, do it properly: head up, shoulders back, toes pointed straight ahead, your bended knee a bit ahead of the rest of your body so that you come down on your full foot, *not* with the weight on your heels as so many of us learned to walk. The proper stride tones up the muscles better.

Avoid elevators and take the stairs. At home, don't grumble over having to retrieve something from the basement or an upstairs bedroom. Take advantage of these opportunities to tone up.

That's half the job. The other half is a regular period of concentrated exercise.

Set aside a half-hour once or twice a week and work at some regimen hard enough to really rev up your circulation. It can be an aerobics class, laps around a swimming pool, or a tough tennis game. It doesn't even have to be something athletic. How about a tango class or a folk dancing club?

The particular activity doesn't matter, as long as it's something you enjoy and it provides an excuse for moving your muscles and getting your pulse rate up to one hundred twenty or whatever your doctor recommends for your physical condition.

Your circulatory system will benefit from head to toe. It's a medical fact that getting the blood to course faster through the blood vessels will float away any small deposits and keep new ones from forming.

Increase the amount of movement in your everyday life and you'll see and feel the advantages very quickly. Your skin will look younger, your figure will be trimmer, and your eyes will sparkle. You'll feel more energetic, and there's a good physiological reason for it: The improvement in circulation that comes from regular exercise means a better oxygen supply. That, coupled with a diet of beauty foods, will increase your vitality and keep you looking younger as the years pass. And, with more oxygen reaching your brain, you'll stay more alert.

Some of the enzymes activated by regular exercise will regulate your appetite naturally, saving you from those sudden cravings that lead you to eat more than you should—and more foolishly than you might otherwise. The other good news is that exercise actually increases your metabolic rate, that is, the speed at which you burn calories. So, if you keep moving you can actually eat more—of the right foods, of course—without gaining weight.

Other enzymes act on your sense of mental well-being, leading you to a feeling of serenity and (the reason there are so many "fitness freaks") almost to a feeling of euphoria. This is the *high* that you get when you are pushing your system to do its best.

Get Enough Sleep

Exercise can slow the aging process, but there is only one activity that allows the body to actually regenerate itself and that is sleep. Sleep is our only opportunity for total physical and mental relaxation.

Skimp and you'll show it. Scientists who study this subject report that you lose as much as 15 percent of your physical and mental capacity if you don't get enough sleep. Few after-midnight galas are going to be worth sacrificing that much of what makes you as good as you are.

But just how much sleep is enough? It varies from one day to the next and from one individual to another. Five hours and one woman is ready to fight tigers, while another is sluggish after eight and a half hours of deep slumber. Listen to what your own body is telling you. If you need more than the average, allow time for it. Don't let yourself be influenced by those who just think you're being lazy.

The time you choose to go to bed and wake up will dictate the amount of time you spend sleeping, but a lot of other habits will determine whether the hours in between are actually restful. Prepare for sleep the way you prepare for any other important segment of your day. Get ready by easing out of the cares of the day and relaxing. Stimulants have to be avoided well before bedtime. So do the problems of business and your personal life. You simply can't keep yourself hyped up until 11:30 working on your presentation for tomorrow's meeting and expect to drop off to dreamland at midnight.

Read a soothing book, or watch something mindless on television for half an hour before getting into bed. Or soak in a warm tub scented with your favorite fragrance. Or sip a glass of warm milk. The U.S. Public Health Service reports new research that shows that a particular piece of grandmotherly advice was well-founded: milk has a high concentration of L-tryptophan, the amino acid that triggers the biochemical process of sleep.

After you've had a good night's sleep, it's equally important not to get up on the wrong side of the bed. Whether you're a morning person, or can't stand to get out of bed until the sun is high in the sky, it's nice to wake up slowly and gently. Stretch while you're still in bed, and then again when you're on your feet. Go over to the window and breathe in the fresh air. You'll feel much more alert and look better as well.

Then help yourself to a glass of warm water into which you've squeezed the juice of half a lemon and added a level teaspoon of honey. All that vitamin C is wonderful for youthful skin and a healthy immune system. In addition, the citric acid does wonders for the circulation in your capillaries. In the long run, it all means more oxygen, which speeds up regeneration of skin cells. Warm lemon juice also gently activates your digestive system and helps to prevent constipation.

You might like to start some days with Vitamin Start, a combination of yoghurt, dried apricots that have soaked overnight in water, and slivered almonds. It's another skin beautifier, full of vitamins A, B, and C.

Fight Stress

Besides the deep sleep of nighttime, you have to set aside some other time of the day to shut out the tensions of your life. Otherwise, the pressures will get to you. Long-term stress takes an enormous toll on your whole body. We say we are *nervous,* but what we are really describing is a wide range of very real physical reactions to the demands placed on us as mothers, daughters, lovers, employees, and neighbors, at virtually every waking moment. And these demands work against our natural beauty.

"Stress born of the cares of daily living can truly wreak havoc on the skin," warns Dr. Jonathan Zizmor, chief of dermatology at St. Vincent's Hospital in New York; "Our emotions aren't just pinned on our collective sleeves; they're literally branded on the flesh!" Dr. Zizmor calls the skin "a window into the individual's inner condition," and maintains, "Many people who come to the doctor seeking explanations of rashes, pimples, or hives actually are often suffering from nothing more than stress, tension, and psychological unhappiness."

In the long run, doing the things that will make you healthy and beautiful—eating right, getting enough exercise, sleeping long enough each night—give you the strength to counteract stress too. But in the short run—in other words, when the events of the day threaten to gobble you up *right now*, set aside some time for yourself. I find that ten minutes will do it, if you really concentrate on yourself for that amount of time. My regimen:

- Sit—or, even better, lie down—in a darkened room, where you are sure you will not be disturbed.

- Close your eyes and try to make your mind totally blank. You can do this easily by repeating one word over and over in your mind. Any word or phrase will do, but pick one with a pleasant sound and no strong connotations. *Lilac looms* is fine, but something on your afternoon shopping list or the name of the project you are about to pick up won't work.

- Then concentrate on relaxing your entire body, one part at a time. Start with your feet and work upwards, really concentrating on how the muscles feel, how the skin feels. If you do it right, you'll feel warm and heavy.

- Then get up slowly and take three deep breaths, inhaling and exhaling slowly.

I try to work in that six-hundred-second routine *before* my body demands it; midday seems to be best. It's really just a matter of good pacing. But, whenever you take this relaxation break, rest assured that you will get up invigorated, your mind and body responding to the pick-me-up with renewed energy for the rest of the day.

The Five-Day Plan

Your very best intentions to *Eat Yourself Beautiful* and improve your lifestyle can go astray. And after a long, sedentary winter, or a period of more stress than usual, or when you've gone out and indulged once too often, your body and state of mind will be in need of revitalization.

How can you rid yourself of the blahs and the fatigue that you haven't been able to shake, lose a few pounds, and see your skin glow again? And how can you do all of these quickly?

In order to explain how you can bring about this amazing transformation of your inner well-being and your outer appearance, we'll talk about the basics of the Five-Day Plan.

The plan provides your system with the unique ability to be its own "detox" unit. During these five days, you can rid yourself of all the toxins that have accumulated over a number of months. The bad effects of all the no-nos—coffee, alcohol, nicotine and tar, fats, and refined sugar and salt—will be eliminated by your system.

Your body's only task will be to process raw vegetables and fruits that contain loads of vitamins and minerals. These, together with all the fiber, liquid, and enzymes that also occur in these foods, will promote the detoxification process while helping to burn off excess pounds as well. The crudités that you'll eat will provide your body with vitamins and minerals that you might have been missing; they will also restore the chemical balance of your skin making you radiant again.

For years, a diet of raw vegetables and fruit has been the basis of the most effective revitalization and purification methods practiced worldwide. As anyone who has ever done this "detox" program can tell you, there's no doubt about the beauty and health potential of these foods.

Raw vegetables and fruit accelerate our metabolism, which means that our digestion is revved up and toxins are eliminated rapidly. The oxygen supply to all the cells is improved and that alone gives you more energy and makes you able to do more. Since you won't be taking in any toxins—coffee, alcohol, fats, or the other beauty no-nos—during these five days, there'll be nothing to prevent you from having the full purifying and revitalizing benefits of the vitamins, minerals, enzymes, and fiber.

Details

We'll tell you what the plan involves on a day-by-day basis for breakfast, lunch, and dinner. Of course, you can switch lunch and dinner. In between you can eat as many crudités as you like (but no avocados because of their high fat content). You can have carrots, cucumbers, celery sticks, cabbage and lettuce leaves, radishes, and tomatoes whenever you like, either in the form of "rabbit food" or liquefied into juice.

You can eat one apple a day, whenever you like. And you can have as much mineral water and herb tea as you like, with lemon or with a daily total of two ounces of skim milk. It's best not to have honey during the five days, but you can use small quantities of artificial sweetener. Coffee, strong tea, and alcohol are definitely out, but you might try a caffeine-free coffee substitute.

More Details

Exercise is terribly important on the Five-Day Plan. Try to exercise for thirty minutes daily during the five days. As a supplement to proper nutrition, exercise is the best route to a vital and youthful body and peace of mind. Regular physical exercise, which gives you an aerobic workout for at least twenty minutes and raises your pulse rate the proper amount for your age and fitness level, has countless beneficial health and beauty effects.

First, the oxygen-carrying capacity of the blood is increased, and, second, blood flows through our bodies faster. These two factors greatly improve the oxygen supply to every organ in our bodies.

And then there's the stepped-up metabolism. Exercise makes us produce more energy, which is burned up faster. That makes for increased vitality and performance in our day-to-day life. Regular exercise gives you the energy and stamina to counter everyday stress.

Your revved up metabolism also accelerates the digestive process and the efficient elimination of toxins. So if you eat fairly well, trying to avoid most toxins, and exercise regularly several times a week, your body will be able to eliminate all the undesirable materials quickly. The resulting improved circulation will supply every part of your body with lots of oxygen, which in turn produces faster cell regeneration, and all of which will be reflected in youthful and glowing skin.

The symptoms of our modern society, such as overweight, constipation, circulatory disturbances, and heart problems, are caused for the most part by poor nutrition and too little exercise. In other words, these are symptoms your body is taking in lots of toxins and is unable to shed them because of a lack of high-fiber nutrition and regular exercise which stimulates the metabolism. Therefore, the toxins remain in our tissues and organs and slow down our circulation and metabolism, which hampers our cellular regeneration. Continuing these bad habits makes our bodies age prematurely. Our lungs lose their capacity to take in large quantities of oxygen. Our muscles lose their tone and, without enough oxygen, they atrophy. And because our skin loses its efficient blood supply, it becomes thin and full of wrinkles and looks old.

If you follow the five-day revitalization plan several times a year, your body can rid itself of its accumulated toxins and undergo a regenerative process. Raw vegetables purify your digestive system and restore your chemical balance (which is upset by the hyperacidity of a "civilized diet" that includes the no-nos). That rebalancing will give you all the good metabolic and circulatory effects that we've been talking about.

Your program of good nutrition and regular exercise (in the form of brisk walking, swimming, tennis, jogging or gymnastics, aerobic dancing, or whatever you enjoy most) needs two more supplements—relaxation and adequate sleep.

During the next five days, try and be in bed by 10 P.M. so that you'll get enough sleep. In addition, try to lie down and relax for at least thirty minutes each day. This shouldn't keep you from spending the rest of your time in a very active way. You're just providing your body with the rest it needs for full revitalization. A tired and stressed organism just can't relax properly. When you've slept enough, you have 15 percent more stamina than when you have too little sleep. In connection with good nutrition and enough exercise, adequate sleep—when your body is sufficiently relaxed to regenerate its forces—really can "keep you young." Your skin will be youthful, your eyes will glow, and your entire body will feel vital and energetic. That's why it's called "beauty sleep."

The best evidence of the amazing effects of the Five-Day Plan comes when you've completed it. You won't need any further persuasion.

But before you do start, check with your doctor; that's an absolute must. While the plan does nothing but good for most people, it's definitely not intended as a substitute for needed medical treatment. If you're already on a special diet, that shouldn't be tampered with either. So, again, NO FIVE-DAY PLAN WITHOUT YOUR DOCTOR'S OKAY.

Try to start the plan on a Thursday if you can. That way you can really take advantage of Friday night, Saturday, and Sunday for your beautification program. The plan will continue through Monday; you can resume your usual beauty foods on Tuesday. In order to reaccustom your body gradually to its usual diet, try to eat mostly raw vegetables for the next four days, but add whole-grain bread; brown rice; whole-grain cereals; a little meat; and of course lots of cooked vegetables, fruit, and fruit juices.

This will enable your body to make full use of the revitalizing action of the Five-Day Plan.

The Evening Before

On the evening before you start the plan (Wednesday), eat very little meat and few carbohydrates, but have a large mixed salad. Don't drink any alcohol. This prepares your system for the purifying effect of the first day.

Thursday (First Day)

Right after you get up, slowly sip a glass of warm water with the juice of half a lemon squeezed into it. This wakes up your system in the most natural way.

BREAKFAST. Two tablespoons of wheat bran mixed with two tablespoons of low-fat yoghurt. With this, eat an apple, pear, or grapefruit.

Forty percent of wheat bran is fiber, which is eliminated by your body in unchanged form. But because of the volume and expanding capacity of the fiber, it activates your digestive system. So your "detox" program starts off with breakfast. It's very important to drink a lot so that the bran can expand properly; try to have two to three cups of liquid. Because of the fiber and liquid it contains, fruit also helps to activate your digestive system. Besides that it gives you vitamin C (especially if you've decided to eat grapefruit), vitamin A, and that important beauty mineral, potassium. Have lots of herb tea with lemon or coffee substitute with some of your daily milk ration for breakfast. No sugar, please! A little artificial sweetener is okay. And you can have as much mineral or tap water as you like. Breakfast is the same all five days; just have a different fruit. Between breakfast and lunch, you can nibble on crudités (except for avocados); there's really no limit on these. And you can eat your daily apple, but nothing more than that for now.

LUNCH. For lunch, there's a crisp and appetizing tossed salad consisting of cucumbers, watercress, tomatoes, onions, leaf lettuce, and two chopped walnuts. The salad contains beauty vitamins A, C, E, F, and the B complex, and beauty minerals calcium, copper, chromium, iodine, iron, magnesium, manganese, potassium, selenium, sulfur, and zinc. (Just the walnuts by themselves contain the vitamin B complex and vitamin F, as well as calcium, copper, iron, magnesium, manganese, and zinc.) The beauty effects of this salad are concentrated on your skin and hair. Vitamin F and iodine will make it lustrous and strong. Have the salad with the *Citrusssssss* dressing and a thin slice of whole-grain bread.

You can have as much salad as you like, but try not to eat so much that you feel uncomfortably full. Between lunch and dinner, have more crudités if you want them, and unlimited amounts of herb tea, coffee substitute, mineral water, and fruit juices, but nothing other than that.

DINNER. In the evening, there's tomato salad with onions and watercress, and vinaigrette dressing containing only one tablespoon of olive oil. With this you can eat two slices of whole-grain flat bread or a thin slice of whole-grain bread.

The tomato salad contains vitamins B_1, B_2, C, and E, and the minerals calcium, chromium, iodine, iron, manganese, potassium, selenium, and sulfur. It's especially good for unlined, supple skin. In addition to fiber, whole-grain bread contains lots of the vitamin B complex and vitamin E, and calcium, copper, iron, manganese, potassium, and zinc. The B vitamins are especially important for beautiful skin and glistening hair.

For dessert, you can have some grapes (about eight ounces) or any other fruit except bananas. Remember that you can have herb tea, coffee substitute, and vegetable juice whenever you want them.

Try to go to sleep early so that your body can take full advantage of the good things you're doing for it.

Friday (Second Day)

The first good thing you can do for your body is to wake up slowly and gently. Take lots of time to stretch, take a few deep breaths in front of an open window, and sip your lemon potion.

Breakfast is the same as Thursday: two tablespoons of wheat bran with two tablespoons of low-fat yoghurt; one piece of fruit (apple, pear, or grapefruit); and herb tea, coffee substitute, or mineral water.

Between breakfast and lunch, you may have lots of the permitted beverages and crudités.

Second-day lunch is the Flowering Orange, which consists of cabbage, an orange, almonds, leeks, and lamb's lettuce. With it, have a yoghurt dressing made of two tablespoons low-fat yoghurt, two tablespoons of vinegar, one tablespoon of fresh orange juice, and herbal seasoning and pepper to taste.

The Flowering Orange gives you vitamins A, C, E, and some of the vitamin B complex. It's really great for clear, smooth skin that looks youthful and resists blemishes.

Accompany the Flowering Orange with a slice of whole-grain flat bread and lots of mineral water.

Your between-meal snack will be your choice of raw vegetables. You might try to take a nap right after lunch and follow that with an exercise period, thirty minutes to an hour, depending on what you're doing.

For this evening, Beauty Greens made up of radicchio, Bibb lettuce, watercress, and half an avocado, with any one of the beauty dressings. Accompany it with a thin slice of whole-grain bread.

Beauty Greens provide you with vitamins A, C, E, and K and B_1 and B_2 members of the vitamin B complex. These are essential for glowing skin and they also prevent blemishes.

If you're not hungry, you can have a smaller salad and skip the bread. You can eat as little or as much as you'd like, and you can even eat only one or two meals. But you should never go hungry!

Saturday (Third Day)

Saturday is fruit day!

Your breakfast is the same as on the two previous days. Between meals please stick to crudités and only limited fruit.

For lunch and dinner, there's a mixed fruit salad with any combination of fruit that you find appealing (except bananas). You can have as much fruit salad as you want but try not to overeat.

Fresh fruit contains vitamin A and large quantities of vitamin C (especially citrus fruits and blueberries), as well as chromium, magnesium, phosphorus, potassium, and lots of fiber and enzymes. These will rev up your metabolism and accelerate elimination of toxins.

Go to bed early again this evening, but don't worry if you're not really tired and don't fall asleep immediately. What's happening is that your system is beginning to recover after three days of beauty foods.

Sunday (Fourth Day)

Sunday is a very pleasant, low-key day. You can sleep as late as you like, and then just relax all day long, read all those sections of the newspaper you never have time for, putter (if you enjoy it), anything that seems like fun. You can play some favorite sport and take a few mild exercise breaks (breathing exercises, easy floor exercises, yoga, etc.).

For lunch, it's Protein Plus, which is made up of Bibb lettuce, radicchio, Boston lettuce, lamb's lettuce, watercress, leeks, and a hard-boiled egg. Have your Protein Plus with vinaigrette dressing (containing only one tablespoon of olive oil) and a slice of whole-grain toast. Drink lots of mineral water from your prettiest glass.

Protein Plus provides you with beauty vitamins A, B$_1$ and B$_2$, D, E, and K as well as the minerals calcium, chromium, iodine, iron, manganese, potassium, selenium, sulfur, and zinc. It has everything you need for strong, healthy hair and nails and beautiful skin.

For supper, have Pink Blush, which contains beets, apples, onions, and dill. The dressing for Pink Blush consists of low-fat yoghurt, vinegar, orange juice, herbal seasoning, and pepper. Omit bread with this one.

Pink Blush contains vitamins A, B$_1$ and B$_2$, C, E, F, and K as well as calcium and potassium. This is very effective in the prevention or management of dry skin and dull, brittle hair. It's also great for your teeth.

Have some herbal tea with lemon and a little artificial sweetener as a pre-bedtime drink.

Monday (Fifth Day)

All good things must come to an end, and that goes for the Five-Day Plan as well. You'll feel and look better and your attitude will be relaxed and refreshed.

Now that you're ready to make use of all that renewed energy and get back to your normal schedule, here's the menu for the last day.

Breakfast is still the same, consisting of two tablespoons of wheat bran mixed with two tablespoons of low-fat yoghurt and an apple, a pear, or a grapefruit. Drink herb tea, coffee substitute, or mineral water.

These beverages together with lots of raw vegetable snacks are for between meals.

For lunch, a variation of the Sunny Salad. This time it's made of an apple, carrots, cabbage, and one-quarter cup of goat cheese and garnished with one level tablespoon of chopped nuts (no raisins). Mix the salad with Citrusssssss dressing, and have it with a thin slice of whole-grain bread and lots of mineral water.

Sunny Salad provides you with vitamin A, the vitamin B complex, and vitamins C, D, E, F, and K (all the ones you need to *Eat Yourself Beautiful*). You'll also have a number of minerals—calcium, chromium, iodine, iron, manganese, magnesium, phosphorus, potassium, selenium, sulfur, and zinc as well as lots of fiber (especially in the carrots and cabbage). Your skin, hair, eyes, and nails will have all the vitamins and minerals they need to look their best.

To finish the Five-Day Plan, your evening meal is a small portion of Hairglow (because you shouldn't eat too much before going to bed). This is made with Chinese cabbage, pear, one chopped walnut, watercress, and one level tablespoon of cottage cheese. Enjoy your Hairglow with low-fat vinaigrette and one slice of whole-grain flatbread.

Hairglow contains lots of vitamin A, as well as the B vitamins and C, D, E, F, and K. There's also calcium, manganese, phosphorus, sulfur, and zinc, everything you need to make your hair gleam and your nails strong.

Go to bed early and the next morning you'll see a beautiful and revitalized you.

As I said in the introduction to the Five-Day Plan, your revitalization program will be all the more effective if you still eat lots of raw vegetables for the next four or five days and avoid alcohol, tobacco, and very fatty and sweet foods.

You can certainly eat whole-grain products, brown rice, fish, poultry, and fruit, as well as fruit juices, low-fat milk, and low-fat yoghurt.

By allowing your body to return to its normal eating pattern gradually, you'll have gotten the maximum beauty and health benefits from the Five-Day Plan.

The Five-Day Plan When You're Away from Home

If you eat out while you're on the plan, you don't have to follow the suggested menus to the letter. Just order a mixed salad or crudité plate and ask for fat-free vinaigrette dressing. You can eat a slice of whole-grain bread, and drink mineral water and you'll still be adhering to the plan.

Lunch at the office is easy too. Just take a little time in the morning to pack your salad with separate dressing. Add a plastic container of raw vegetables for snack time, take along a few herbal teabags, and you're set.

Dr. de Winter's QUESTIONNAIRE AND GUIDE TO A HEALTHY LIFESTYLE

Your Diet

Answer yes or no to the following.

1. Do you like to eat at least one three-course meal a day?
2. Do you add sugar to food or drink?
3. Do you eat chocolate regularly?
4. Do you have butter every day?
5. Do you eat a lot of cheese?
6. Do you have cream with dessert, coffee or tea, or fruit?
7. Do you buy whole milk rather than skim?
8. Do you eat more than four eggs a week?
9. Do you eat meat without trimming the fat first?
10. Do you have fried food more than twice a week?
11. Do you eat meat more than twice a week?
12. Do you add salt when you cook?
13. Do you always salt the food on your plate?
14. Do you eat convenience foods more than twice a week?
15. Do you eat white bread?
16. Are you addicted to some foods?
17. Do you drink more than four cups of coffee a day?
18. Do you drink more than four cups of tea a day?
19. Do you drink fewer than four eight-ounce glasses of water a day?
20. Do you think vegetables are boring to eat?
21. Do you eat fruit only infrequently?

Your Body

1. Are you weight conscious?
2. Have you kept your figure trim?
3. Do you try to raise your pulse rate every day by exercise?
4. Would you walk or run upstairs rather than take the elevator?
5. Do you make a real effort to be fit?
6. Do you feel unhappy when deprived of exercise?
7. Do you smoke fewer than six cigarettes a week?
8. Do you drink fewer than two alcoholic drinks a day?
9. Do you eat at least two tablespoons of bran a day?
10. Is whole-grain cereal one of the main items on your shopping list?
11. Do you have regular bowel movements?
12. Do you avoid using laxatives?
13. Do you have a medical checkup regularly?
14. Do you have regular pelvic examinations and pap smears?
15. Do you examine your breasts often for lumps and other changes?

Your Personality

1. Do you lack confidence?
2. Do you feel that there's not much fun in your life?
3. Are you confused about your goals?
4. Is your work boring?
5. Do you suffer from feelings of hopelessness?
6. Do you panic before an important assignment?
7. Do you have butterflies in your stomach throughout it?
8. Do you fail to do yourself justice on a regular basis?
9. Do you feel exhausted after making a special effort?
10. Do you get impatient when delayed by anything or anyone?
11. Do you often try to do two things at the same time?
12. Do you feel guilty when you're not doing something constructive?
13. Do you find it difficult to relax when you're on your own?
14. Do you crave recognition?
15. Are you overly competitive?
16. Do you refuse to admit failure?
17. Do you think you work harder than most people?

18. Are you easily discouraged?
19. Are you afraid of cancer?
20. Are you ultra-sensitive?
21. Do you bottle up your feelings?
22. Do you harbor grudges?
23. Are you often depressed?
24. Do you take tranquilizers?
25. Do you take antidepressants?
26. Do you take sleeping pills?
27. Do you take painkillers regularly?

Under Stress

If the person closest to you died, would you:
1. Be able to express your grief?
2. Feel you had lost the only person you ever really related to?
3. Feel that no one would ever love you again?
4. Feel that you could never cope on your own?
5. Expect the loss to ruin your life completely?

If you were fired, would you feel:
1. Helpless and hopeless?
2. That your self-confidence had been destroyed?
3. That your faith in the world had been undermined?
4. Powerless to change the situation?
5. Completely useless and unemployable?
6. Suicidal?

If you had broken off a relationship with your partner because of his infidelity, would you feel:
1. Bitter and vengeful?
2. Unable to go out and meet people?
3. Wracked with guilt?
4. Regretful of the past?
5. Full of hate for the other woman?
6. Full of hate for him?

Scoring

Your ability to stay healthy depends on what we *eat*, how we *think*, and how much we *move*. Your response to the above questions should indicate in which of these areas you are most vulnerable. In section one, *Your Diet*, score one point for every *no* answer. In section two, *Your Body*, score one point for every *yes*. In sections three and four, *Your Personality* and *Under Stress*, score one point for every *no*.

LESS THAN 30:
You are putting yourself seriously at risk by your uncontrolled eating habits, lack of will power, and refusal to take any interest in your health. You find it hard to assert yourself and take control of your life, and the resulting stress and nervous tension threaten your immune system and make you vulnerable to illness. Unhappiness and frustration also drive you to eat and drink too much. This in turn makes you sluggish and overweight, which makes you want to avoid exercise. Yours is a formula for disaster. Act now to change your bad habits. Give up smoking, cut down on alcohol, radically change your diet, and take up yoga and regular exercise. It's not too late, but you are the only one who can do it.

30–60:
Your score indicates a variety of minor sins scattered throughout these three vital areas of your life, or a major weakness in one—go back and see where you lost points. Your emotional life is not unhappy, but you find it hard to stay on an even keel. In your periodic ups and downs you seek comfort in eating and indulge yourself in the wrong kinds of food. You also have a tendency to worry and depression, feeling tapped or in a rut. In better times you are capable of turning over a new leaf and rediscovering your interest in your health, figure, and appearance. Decide now to stick to your plan for a sensible diet, more exercise, and better balance in your life. Concentrate on positive thinking and slow but steady progress toward your goals. Don't give in to depression or morbid thoughts, which make you more susceptible to illness.

60–80:
Your wide-ranging knowledge of health matters and your awareness of your body are reflected in this high score. You have developed a high degree of motivation and self-control, avoiding or restricting all sugar, fats, salt, and red meat in your diet. You drink very little alcohol and never smoke. Emotionally you possess an unusual degree of resilience and stability, but you also make the effort to organize your life to eliminate as much overwork and stress as possible. In addition, your life plan includes regular exercise and opportunities for relaxation. Your prospects for staying healthy are excellent.

Practical Hints

1. Don't eat meat or fried food more than once a week.
2. Make fresh, unpeeled vegetables and whole-grain cereal the major part of every meal.
3. Add two to three tablespoons of bran to your food every day.
4. Avoid butter, cream, and whole milk.
5. Eat more fish.
6. At most, drink two glasses of wine every day.
7. Avoid sugar.
8. Drink two glasses of water in the morning to help prevent constipation.
9. Never take elevators; walk up stairs instead.
10. Take up yoga or meditation.
11. Use a barrier method of contraception.
12. Never have intercourse with a man suffering from genital warts or herpes.
13. Be discriminating in your choice and number of sexual partners.
14. Report any lump or discharge to your doctor *immediately.*

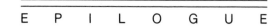

E   P   I   L   O   G   U   E

The degree to which we can enjoy life depends mainly on our peace of mind and the good health of such bodily functions as vision, hearing, intellect, appetite, digestion, and mobility. Heeding the recommendations in this book will go a long way toward insuring good health and a boundless vitality and zest for living.

The average person would prefer not to have to work for good health, but without effort, it cannot be achieved. Elementary rules must be obeyed, and the principal one of these, which is repeated throughout the book, is that all eating habits must be simple, regular, moderate, and wholesome. In fact, the quality of our lives hinges far more on how much we allow our bodies to degenerate—as a result of habitually harmful habits—than it depends on our actual ages. When our tissues degenerate and lose their youthfulness and elasticity, this is not a result of the aging process. Rather, we grow old because we make them degenerate by our unhealthy living habits. By contrast, a well-functioning, oxygen-rich bloodstream, generated by sensible eating habits and regular exercise, will keep our bodies healthy and fresh, thus enhancing our capability for continued fitness and beauty.

In other words, early adoption of the dietary discretion and restraint recommended in this book as a way of life, coupled with regularly sustained exercise, will insure a rare sense of inner harmony and self-confidence. And this harmony and self-confidence are reflected in a more healthy and beautiful you.

Anyone anxious to avoid many of today's countless dietary pitfalls would do well to pay attention to the especially helpful and practical tips that give the reader a wide variety of health-promoting alternatives. This is particularly helpful because we have learned to like food that is richer, softer, and sweeter than ever before. It is richer because we eat more fat; it is softer because it is processed and refined to a high degree and has lost its natural fiber content (together with other necessary nutrients); and it is sweeter because our greatly increased sugar consumption makes us prefer sweet foods, which manufacturers are only too happy to supply. This book is quite explicit about which particular eating habits are harmful and it successfully clarifies a number of old prejudices and misconceptions.

There are about forty substances, all mentioned in the book, that we need to eat for good health and general fitness, but no longer do. Instead, we tend to fill ourselves with refined, high-calorie foods, rich in fat and sugar. Then, as a result of feeling full, we leave out certain substances that the body cannot do without.

Reading this book will make us realize that eating what we like and eating what is healthy are compatible, and that our choice of food also decides our health and our appearance.

In summary, this scientifically sound book shows that it is possible, indeed desirable, to *Eat Yourself Beautiful,* and it tells you how clearly and simply.

Dr. Jan de Winter, MD, FRCR, FFR, RCSI, ADMR

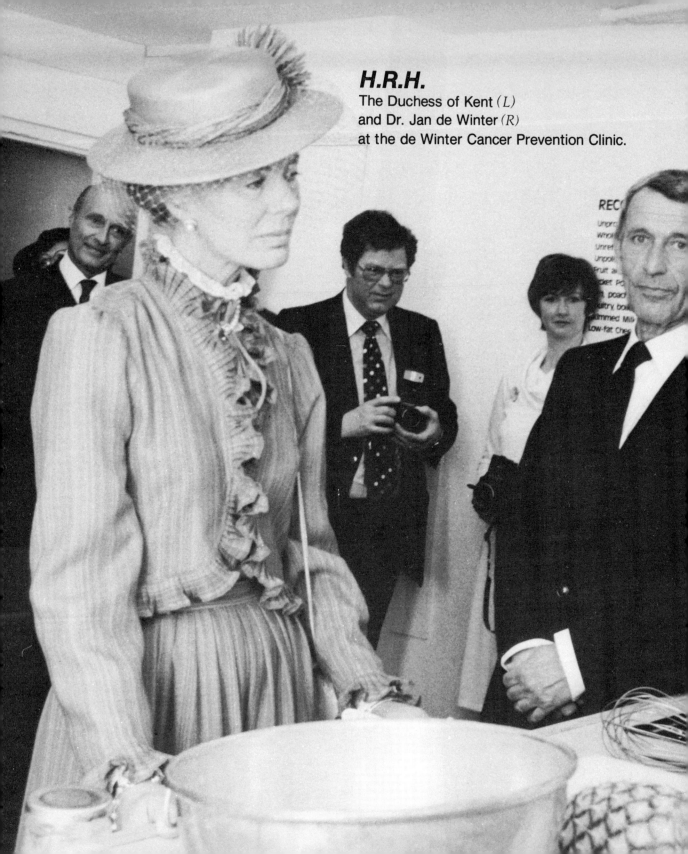

H.R.H.
The Duchess of Kent (L)
and Dr. Jan de Winter (R)
at the de Winter Cancer Prevention Clinic.

Daniele de Winter received her great understanding of the correlation between diet, stress, and disease while working as a dietary assistant in her father, Dr. Jan de Winter's, renowned Clinic for Cancer Prevention Advice (England). This free, walk-in clinic, for which he was awarded the Gold Medal of the National Society for Cancer Relief by the Duchess of Kent, offers health education and a full range of backup facilities. Staffed by over sixty volunteers, including a French chef, yoga experts, aerobic instructors, physicians, and many other professionals integrated within the prevention sciences, the Cancer Advice Clinic serves scores of "healthy" people every day.

After completing an eighty-point questionnaire on diet, stress, exercise, sexual behavior, and addictions, the patient has a thorough interview with Dr. de Winter, in which to ask questions and express concerns. He uncovers the risk factors threatening the patient's long-term well-being and proceeds to correct them. The clinic offers so much support and valuable advice that the patient is able to resist temptations and destructive behavior patterns, without undergoing any additional stress.

Dr. de Winter and his trained staff want to see patients when they are well—so they'll stay that way. As a pioneering cancer specialist who has built an international reputation, he aims to prevent the one out of every four cancer cases that is self-inflicted. Both he and his daughter, Daniele, are indeed living proof of their well-grounded theories.

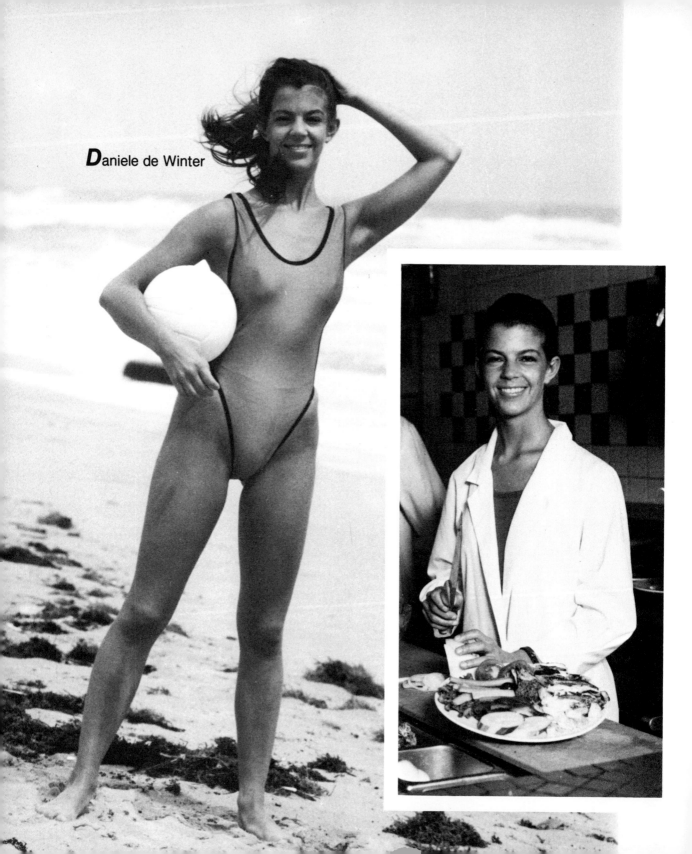

Daniele de Winter

DANIELE DE WINTER grew up in Sussex, England, in a home where, due to her father's medical knowledge, high-fiber foods and low-fat cheeses were bywords, while cigarettes, alcohol, and chocolates were virtually unknown. Having successfully completed her A-level examinations, she moved to Vienna to study graphic art. After receiving her diploma, Daniele began working as a jewelry designer in the world-renowned enamel business built up by her mother, Michaela Frey, and pioneered a collection of new geometric jewelry designs. These quickly became bestsellers, giving Daniele a name as one of the new forces to be reckoned with in the field of jewelry design.

Always fascinated by her father's medical research, Daniele has worked as his dietary assistant at the Dr. Jan de Winter Clinic for Cancer Prevention Advice since it was founded in 1982 and has gained great insight into the correlation between diet and disease. In 1984 she wrote her first cookbook, *What the Doctor Ordered*, together with her father. Because of its success in Great Britain, Daniele translated the cookbook into German, and it is now being sold in Austria, Germany, and Switzerland.

Known by her friends as ultrahealthy, Daniele does not drink or smoke, loves to keep very fit, and eats according to the principles she and her father worked out. She is also a part-time model and living proof of the lifestyle she recommends.

DR. JAN DE WINTER studied medicine at the Universities of Prague, Vienna, Berne, and London. Later he became a Fellow of the Royal College of Radiologists in London; a Fellow of the Faculty of Radiologists, Royal College of Surgeons, in Ireland; a Visiting Senior Fellow of the University of Sussex; and the first non-American to be elected a member of The Society of Computed Body Tomography of America. For thirty-one years, between 1950 and 1981, he was the Senior Medical Consultant in charge of cancer treatment at the Royal Sussex County Hospital in Brighton. For the past fifteen years he has made the prevention of nutrition-related cancer his speciality and has published several books and lay guides on the subject: *How to Avoid Cancer* (1981); *How to Die Young at Ninety* (1983); *The Truth About Cancer* (1986); and, with Daniele de Winter, *What the Doctor Ordered* (1984).

In 1982 he opened his own Clinic for Cancer Prevention Advice in the heart of Brighton's shopping district, the first of its kind in Europe. A clinic where all are encouraged to walk in on impulse at any time, without an appointment and while still fit, to find out how to remain healthy. Each person's potential for continued good health is assessed from an eighty-point questionnaire that covers diet, stress, exercise, alcohol habits, cigarette consumption, heredity, sexual behavior, and other related topics. These questions help in identifying the health-undermining risk factors of an individual. These risk factors are then corrected with the help of a full range of back-up facilities, including cooking demonstrations and tasting in the slim-line diet kitchen, psychological consultations and psychotherapy, meditation classes, slimming advice, cervical smear tests, breast self-examination education, and soon, mammography. All of these services are available on the premises and are free of charge.

For his services to cancer sufferers, Dr. de Winter was presented with the Gold Medal of the National Society for Cancer Relief in 1981 by the Duchess of Kent and was elected its President for

Life. In 1985, he was presented with the Evian Award in recognition of his contribution to the health of the nation by the Duke of Gloucester. At the international film festival in Bucharest, in 1985, he won an award for his film on the Clinic for Cancer Prevention Advice and its aims. Finally, he has been selected by the Board of the International Biographical Centre, Cambridge, England, for special mention in the dedication section of its Dictionary's 1986 edition, as one of its most distinguished honorees.

His teaching, now generally accepted, is that cancer and health, like fire and water, are incompatible and, being mutually exclusive, cannot coexist. It follows that cancer and other similarly degenerative diseases such as heart disease, high blood pressure, stroke, diabetes, and arthritis should be avoidable through the conscientious maintenance of health—that is, through a strict adherence to a sensible diet—because there is a vital link among nutrition, overweight, and the avoidance of degenerative diseases. We know, for instance, that six million Americans who are alive today will die of bowel cancer because they cannot resist the temptation to overeat. Apart from looking less attractive and running a serious risk of degenerative disease, an obese person has the added disadvantage of aging more rapidly. The reason for this is simple: We are as old as our arteries, and the condition of our arteries hinges on the degree of self-imposed moderation and restraint. When our tissues degenerate, they do not degenerate because we grow old; we grow old because we make them degenerate by living in an unhealthy way.

There are several misconceptions that need to be corrected. We assume, wrongly, that it is normal for old people to lose their mobility and energy; to suffer rheumatism, arthritis, and to have difficulty in breathing; to become overweight; and to lose some of their alertness. Nothing could be further from the truth. Similarly, and again wrongly, we accept cancer and heart disease as part of our normal lives; they certainly don't need to be.

Beauty Books

Alive with Color!, Easy, Sophisticated Color Analysis, by Leatrice Eiseman
ISBN 87491-522-X/$18.95 hardcover/Beauty, 250 pages, 8 × 9, 36 pages full color.

Always in Style, Your Shape, Your Style, by Doris Pooser
ISBN 87491-785-9/$16.95 hardcover/Beauty, 200 pages, 8 × 9, illustrated throughout, 40 full color photographs, black and white (including 6 seasonal color flowcharts), 60 illustrations.

Big & Beautiful, How to be Gorgeous on Your Own Grand Scale, by Ruthanne Olds
ISBN 87491-725-5/$8.95 quality paper/Beauty,
ISBN 87491-088-9/$16.95 hardcover/Beauty, 200 pages, 8 × 9, 12 pages full color.

Color Me Beautiful, Updated!, Discover Your Natural Beauty through Color, by Carole Jackson. The original seasonal color classic! 30-color palettes for Winters, Springs, Summers & Autumns.
ISBN 87491-756-5/$14.95 hardcover/Beauty, 212 pages, 24-page color section, b/w illus.

Eat Yourself Beautiful Your Strategy for Lifelong Beauty, by Daniele de Winter
ISBN 87491-860-X/$12.95 quality paperback/Beauty & Health, 184
pages, 8 × 9, color photographs, illustrations, recipes, index.

8 Minute Makeovers, Your Most Beautiful Face for Every Occasion, by
Clare Miller
ISBN 87491-736-0/$15.95 hardcover/Beauty, 172 pages, 8 × 9, 12 full-
color pages.

8 Moves to a Perfect Body, Shrink a Size in 3 Weeks without Dieting, by
Sheri Blair, photographs by Lisa Berg
ISBN 87491-727-1/$4.95 quality paper/Health, 96 pages, $5^1/2 × 8^1/2$,
photographs throughout.

El Color de Tu Belleza, por Carole Jackson. Now it's in Spanish! It's the same
212 colorful pages selling for $9.95 in quality paperback.
ISBN 87491-770-0/$9.95 quality paperback/Beauty, 212 pages,
$7^1/2 × 8^1/4$, 24 page color section, b/w illus.

Make the Most of Your Child's Good Looks, For children 5–12 and teens 13–18,
boys and girls!, by Anne Schwab
ISBN 87491-861-8/$12.95 quality paperback/Beauty, 172 pages, 8 × 9,
12 color pages, illustrated throughout.

Image Consulting: the NEW Career, How to Build an Exciting Money-Making
Career on Your Own Time, by Joan Timberlake
ISBN 87491-728-X/$8.95 quality paper/Careers, 150 pages, 8 × 9, index.

New Image for Women: The Fashion Academy's Official Guide for Personal
Image Development, by Gerrie Pinckney, President and Executive
Director, The Fashion Academy
ISBN 87491-863-4/$18.95 quality hc /Beauty & Fashion, 192 pages,
$8^1/2 × 10^1/2$, 75 color plates with color palettes, fully illustrated.

Waiting In Style, By Alyson Fendel. A maternity wardrobe that works
ISBN 87491-553-8/$14.95 hardcover,
ISBN 87491-702-6/$9.95 quality paper.

The Winner's Style, The Modern Male's Passport to Perfect Grooming, by
Kenneth J. Karpinski, Foreword by Doris Pooser
ISBN 87491-824-3/$9.95 quality paper/Men's Fashion/196 pages, 36
color plates, illustrated throughout, glossary, appendices, index.

Your Colors at Home, Decorating with Your Seasonal Colors, by Lauren Smith
& Rose Bennett Gilbert
ISBN 87491-748-4/$18.95 hardcover/Home Decorating, 200 pages, 30

color plates and illustrations, 4 seasonal color palettes with 40 decorating colors each, 40 photographs and illustrations.

Your Medical Image, Making It Work for You, by Carole Mosbacher
ISBN 87491-857-X/$25.00 looseleaf bound/Image consulting.

Find Your Seasoning Find Yourself, The Herbopsychiatric Approach to Riches, Sex, Diet & Success, by Robert Hickey, Hp.D. & Kathleen Hughes, Hp.D. A spoof on all categorical self-help books. Nominated by England's *Bookseller* magazine as the most ludicrous book of the year!
ISBN 87491-759-X/$5.95 quality paper/Humor, 96 pages, 6 × 9, b/w illustrations throughout.

INDEX